AF560031

Hospital Administration System

Hospital Administration System

C. Charles

ANMOL PUBLICATIONS PVT. LTD.
NEW DELHI - 110 002 (INDIA)

ANMOL PUBLICATIONS PVT. LTD.

H.O.: 4374/4B, Ansari Road, Darya Ganj
New Delhi-110 002 (India)
Ph.: 23278000, 23261597
B.O.: 1015, Ist Main Road, BSK IIIrd Stage
IIIrd Phase, IIIrd Block
Bangalore - 560 085 (Karnataka)
Ph: 080-41723429, Tel/Fax: 080-2672 3604
Visit us at: www.anmolpublications.com

Hospital Administration System

First Published, 2008

ISBN 978-81-261-3284-3

PRINTED IN INDIA

Printed at Mehra Offset Press, Delhi.

Contents

Preface

Hospital is an institution that provides medical, surgical, or psychiatric care and treatment for the sick or the injured. Administration is a process of direction, overall co-ordination in an agency designed to carry out some agreed purpose with economy and effectiveness in the Hospital. It is the determination and clarification of function, the formulation of policies and procedures, delegation of authority, selection, supervision and training of staffs, mobilization and organization of available and appropriate resources so that the purpose of the Institution may be fulfilled. This book has been designed to provide a platform for all hospital administration experts and others interested in hospital set ups as a science and aims to provide a medium for free and healthy interaction with easy access to relevant information related to inpatient and outpatient registration and admission; online bed allocation; provide complete information about a patient to authorized visitors; provide information regarding package deals for a patient for a fixed cost including company sponsored packages; provide ready information about doctors and staff regarding scheduling and appointments; health cards; insurance; etc. In most hospitals the need of the hour is an in depth study of the existing procedures to streamline them. The current procedures may have been effective when incorporated but since then, the business requirement has changed, the environment has changed, the doctor/patient ratio has changed, the investigating techniques have changed, the surgical procedures have changed and the patient population has exploded. Medical Equipment has become electronic and its output can be interfaced with computers and their software.

Every hospital is unique and has its own peculiar functioning procedures and methodologies. It is therefore necessary to develop software to cater to these requirements. Accordingly a consulting team headed by a project manager will study the requirements, analyze them and then proceed to design an application specific to the organization. For example, the application will be designed with the browser as the front end and oracle 9i as the back end. This gives the most robust design. The entire data is stored and managed in one database. Oracle 9i is the most robust database. With a browser as the front end the client is very thin. The entire data is stored on one server. The hospital can acquire the most economically priced computers for the front end, as they don't need any drives or software to run. A minimal RAM is required. The savings are phenomenal. The system becomes absolutely secure as no data resides on the clients. The moment a user sign's off the node becomes a dud box. The system lends itself to physical security because there is only one server to protect. All the data resides on the server. The client has only adequate software to run a browser. Each user has privileges granted to him/her by the administrator. He may use the system only after logging in and that too only to the extent that is needed by him and allowed to him. This ensures the information is available on a need to know basis. The software is so designed that it protects the system. Once a user has logged out that node cannot provide any information to anyone. *'Breaking in'* is well neighing impossible when we are using oracle 9i. The reception is divided into two windows. One deals with registration of new patients and the other deals with providing help to the visitors. From the time the patient presents himself at the reception desk to the time he is discharged, every activity is recorded through a computer node on to the server. The same information about him, when needed is retrieved through a node from the server. There is no paper trail. The system is a complete wizard for a doctor. Anything that needs to be done for, or to a patient can be ordered, planned and executed from the desktop of the examining doctor, and from one browser window. No new windows are opened and closed. No complicated training is required to use the software. Everything is self-explanatory. At the click of a button a doctor can check the availability of blood in the blood bank for an operation; book an operation theater with entire staff and equipment for an operation; chat with a surgeon to ask him to execute a surgery; admit and book a bed in a ward; order any kind of investigation; read the results of any kind of investigation; read entire clinical history; ask the opinion of another doctor on the case; check availability of medicines; prescribe medicines; enter charges; etc. Following are various major activities performed by hospital administrators:

— Management of Family Medicine OPD, Special OPD and Paying Clinics.

— Posting of various hospital staffs including house officers on daily as well as on monthly basis.

— Provide list of hospital items to procurement section for proper utilization and consumption in various areas of services with the help of departments.

— Management of all in-patient services.

— Supervision and cleanliness of the entire hospital complex.

— Providing and maintaining the hospital information system.

— Management and supervision of all support sections viz. (CSSD, Laundry, MRD, Kitchen etc).
— Helps in the management of Emergency and CLS
— 24 hours Call Duty Officers for various administrative services in hospital.
— Assist in free care services of the hospital.
— Provide counseling to the stressed staffs, patients and relatives.
— Orientation to hospital staffs and students.

This publication entitled "Hospital Administration System" is published specifically to clarify the aforementioned issues and provide options for solutions.

—Editor

1

The Hospital Administration Tool: An Introduction

The Hospital Administration Tool (HAT) provides a graphical interface to manage openadaptor™ object messages (arrays of DataObjects) which have caused an exception as they pass through an Adaptor and have therefore been rejected and collected in a data source called "the hospital". The HAT provides a means of viewing these "failed" messages (patients) and, depending on the security privileges, modify the attributes/structure that caused the problems in the first place. Alternatively, patients can be simply deleted from the hospital.

The HAT comes as an independent standalone application with a swing GUI. As you start the program it loads all adjustable configuration details out of a properties file ("hat.props").

Starting the Hospital Administration Tool

Important: The HAT requires a minimum of JDK 1.2 or later as it is based on the *javax.swing* and *java.awt* packages - it will not run under previous versions of Java.

To resolve all class references you have to add the openadaptor™ libraries to the classpath. HAT expects to find a file "hat.props" accessible in the classpath, so don't forget to add the properties file to a directory accessible by the classpath.

To start HAT, type:

```
java org.openadaptor.hospital.HAT
```

As HAT starts it loads the properties file and displays the Hospital Chooser dialogue box. Once the user has selected the desired hospital and confirms the database connection details the main swing GUI is displayed and the application starts to load entries ("patients") from the "hospital". The number of rows loaded is limited by a parameter defined in the properties file.

To stop the HAT you just have to use the menu item "File->Exit" or close the swing frame.

Logging

As with openadaptor, the HAT is designed to use Log4J as its logger. Out of the box, the default openadadptor formatting will be applied. However, you can supply your own configuration file by including the following in the HAT properties file:

```
log4j.configuration = [path to the config file]
```

Data Sources Supported

There are currently two supported options for storing the patients - in a database or a file. If we use a file, then there is no method of storing the security metadata and the HAT provides a read-only view of the patient data. Depending on the properties set, the HAT automatically configures itself for the appropriate data source:

```
# database settings
HAT.hospitalName.1 = Hospital_A
HAT.dbDriver.Hospital_A = com.sybase.jdbc.SybDriver
```

```
HAT.dbURL.Hospital_A = jdbc:sybase:Tds:localhost:11222
HAT.dbUser.Hospital_A = oa_user
HAT.dbPassword.Hospital_A = oa_password
HAT.dbHospital.Hospital_A = oa_hospital

# file settings
HAT.hospitalName.2 = File_A
HAT.fileName.File_A = /tmp/hospital.dat
```

By default the patients are stored in a file using the internal DataObject XML format. In order to read and interpret this format, the HAT uses the openadaptor™ *org.openadaptor.adaptor.standard.FileSource* component to read in the hospital patients. This means that any specific properties that are supported by the FileSource can also be used by the HAT. For example, you could use the following to specify that they hospital file is of CSV format:

```
HAT.File_A.DOStringReader =
org.openadaptor.dostrings.DelimitedStringReader
HAT.File_A.NumAttributes = 6
HAT.File_A.FieldDelimiter = 44
```

Points to Note

- The format used for the prefix of HAT properties is different to those used for openadaptor properties. This will be sorted out in due time.
- The HAT automatically sets the *InputFileName* property for the FileSource based on the file name passed so it is not necessary to set it in the properties file.
- A read-only view is provided for file based hospitals.

Security

There are three levels of security that can be applied to the HAT:

— hospital database connection: at the most basic of levels, a user must supply a SQL username and password to connect to the Hospital database. These details can be stored in the properties file to provide a rudimentary auto-login feature.

— user roles: once connected to the hospital database, the user is authenticated and its application role determined (see immediately below for details). These determine various application actions and functions that can be performed by the user.

— editable attribute mask: to provide an even more granular level of security, users who have rights to modify a patient's payload can be restricted even further by defining which attributes of a particular DataObject type can be edited. For example, if the hospital contains patients with DataObjects of type "Trade", you may not want anyone to be able to modify the "Bid Amount" attribute.

User Roles

All users are given one of four user roles when they connect to a hospital. These roles determine which of the application features and functions they are permitted to perform. The following roles are defined:

— HATUser - can load patients from the Hospital, validate a patient's payload, clear the Patient List, choose another Hospital to administer

— HATManager - can Validate + Discharge a patient from the Hospital, delete a patient from the Hospital

— HATController - can delete all the loaded patients from the Hospital, admit/re-admit a patient to the Hospital, discharge a patient from the Hospital, add/remove DataObjects to the payload

— HATAdmin - can modify a payload's DataObject and Attributes.

— HATSecurity - can modify the other's users roles as well as the editable attribute mask. This role is designed to be separate from the other roles and should not be used to give access to the hospital patient data itself (i.e. just use this role to administer the users and not to edit the patient data)

As the roles increase they inherit the permissions from the previous role. For example, HATAdmins can perform ALL tasks.

NB: If no role is defined then the user will be given the HATUser role by default which essentially offers a read-only view of the hospital.

Editable Attributes

Users who have been granted permission to modify the patient's payload can be further restricted by defining a map of the individual attributes that can be edited for particular DataObjects. This is basically a mapping between a user role and a DataObject type with a list of the editable attributes. Attributes omitted from this list are read-only. Therefore, if there are no entries for a DataObject type then all its attributes are read-only.

If the list of attributes contains a single value ("EDIT_ALL_ATTRIBUTES") then all attributes for that DataObject type are editable.

Authorisation Method

Currently, the HAT uses SQL usernames, password and security tables in the database to lookup the user's roles and editable attribute details. This will be extended so the information can also be written to a LDAP store. The method used is defined in the properties file:

HAT.authorisationMethod = database

User roles are stored in the DBusMH_UserRole database table. There is a script under the *org.openadaptor.sql* directory that creates this table. This is a relational link table between the DBusMH_User and DBusMH_Role tables. This data should be maintained via the "Admin" menu in the HAT tool. If there is no entry for a specified role then it is assumed that there are no users of that role.

Editable attributes are stored in the DBusMH_EditableAttributes table. There is a script under the *org.openadaptor.sql* directory that creates this table. This is essentially a map of user roles to DataObject types with a list of the attributes that are editable. This is a relational link table between the DBusMH_Attribute and DBusMH_Role tables. These data should be maintained via the "Admin" menu in the HAT tool.

The Menu Bar: The File Menu

File -> Clear Patient List

Clears all the patients loaded into the HAT. This does not delete them from the database.

File -> Load From Hospital

Loads the "oldest" patients from the hospital. The number of patients loaded is limited by a parameter entered in the subsequent message box displayed.

The default value is defined in the HAT properties file. All patients loaded will be inserted to the patient list window with its timestamp. The timestamp indicates the date and time the message has been admitted to the hospital. The progress of the database loading is displayed in the status line.

File -> Choose Hospital

Loads the Hospital Chooser dialogue which allows users to select which hospital to administer.

The list of hospitals in the combo box are defined in the HAT properties file. Each one is identified by an incremental number at the end of the *HAT.hospitalName* attribute. The value for this attribute must be a unique name.

HAT.hospitalName.1 = Hospital_A

HAT.dbDriver.Hospital_A = com.inet.tds.TdsDriver

HAT.dbURL.Hospital_A = jdbc:inetdae:myserver.myorg.com:1434

HAT.dbUser.Hospital_A = oaUser

HAT.dbPassword.Hospital_A = oaPassword

HAT.dbHospital.Hospital_A = oaHospital

HAT.hospitalName.2 = Hospital_B

HAT.dbDriver.Hospital_B = com.inet.tds.TdsDriver

HAT.dbURL.Hospital_B = jdbc:inetdae:myotherserver.myorg.com:1434

HAT.dbUser.Hospital_B = otherUser

HAT.dbPassword.Hospital_B = otherPassword

HAT.dbHospital.Hospital_B = otherHospital

NB: if any of the attributes are missing from the properties file then the Hospital Chooser will not proceed until the user has supplied them manually into the dialogue box.

Once the details have been added satisfactorily to the dialogue, the user can test the database connection by clicking on the appropriate button. This will connect to the database and try to obtain information about the supplied hospital table. An appropriate message is displayed.

Users can also opt to cancel the dialogue which will

either return them to the HAT tool with the current hospital settings intact or if the dialogue was displayed as they started the application then the application exits.

NB: If the application is using database security then the username and password in the right hand side of the dialogue are disabled as these details are the same as the ones in the left hand side.

There are two properties file parameters that effect the way that the patients are loaded from the hospital.

```
HAT.dbRowLimit = 100
HAT.dbSlowLoadLimit = 30
```

HAT.dbRowLimit sets the maximum number of patients to be read in from the database in any one go. This stops the application trying to load 10000 records all at once if the hospital is large.

HAT.dbSlowLoadLimit provides the application with a method of asynchronous database access. Basically, this parameter indicates the number of records that will be fully populated immediately and then the rest will be read in using a background process.

File -> refresh

Reloads the patients from the hospital using the existing load limit parameters.

File -> Exit

Exits the application. The first thing that happens is that the application checks whether there is any unsaved payload changes and prompts the user to save them if necessary. Then, any background loading activities are stopped, the GUI is disposed and the application is terminated.

The GUI

All functionality of HAT is accessible from the swing GUI. From here, particularly from the menu, you can trigger all patient functions.

The GUI contains the following components:

- The pull-Down menu bar
- The patient list window which contains the messages loaded from the hospital. Each patient is displayed with its timestamp
- The patient detail panel. Detail information (Reject reason, application, subject) for the selected patient is displayed here
- The patient payload list. The selected patient can contain one or more DataObjects which will be listed inside this window. The data objects named "SDO 0", "SDO 1",...,"SDO n". SDO means "SimpleDataObject"
- The attribute list. Each DataObject in the current patient's payload contains a set of attributes. Each attribute is made up of a name, value and type.
- Context sensitive popup menus. Depending on the panel, you can click with the right mouse button to have a context sensitive menu brought up. Actions appropriate for the panel you clicked on are displayed

The Patient Menu

Patient -> Validate

Triggers a validation of the selected patient and it's DataObject payload. HAT allows you to define classes that validate a certain DataObject types. To do this you must add a line to the properties file that has a parameter name of [DO type]Validator and a value that is the classpath for this type. For example, if the adaptor is processing "Trade" DataObjects then we would include the following line in the properties file:

TradeValidator = org.myorg.dataobjects.TradeValidator

NB: the validator class must implement the *org.openadaptor.hospital.helpers.HATValidator* interface

In this case, if we are validating a patient whose DataObject type is "Trade" then the application will instantiate the *org.myorg.dataobjects.TradeValidator* and calls its *isValid()* method.

Patient -> Validate + Discharge

Validates the patient as above and then marks it for discharge in the database.

Patient -> Delete From Hospital

Physically deletes the selected patient from the hospital database.

Patient -> Delete All Loaded Patients

Physically deletes ALL the patients loaded into the HAT. This is achieved by taking the timestamps of the first and last patients in the patient list and deleting all patients in the database between them. This is not a great solution as it relies on the original SQL select statement ordering the patients correctly as they are read out of the database in the first place!

Patient -> Discharge

Sets the patient's *Status* field in the hospital database to *DISCHARGE_WAIT*. The HAT does not re-publish patients to the adaptor as there is an AbstractSource class (*org.openadaptor.adaptor.hospital.HospitalSource*) that queries the hospital directly for patients waiting to be discharged and re-publishes them.

Patient -> Reset Status/Admit

Sets the patient's *Status* field in the hospital database to *NEW*.

Patient -> Re-Admit

Set the patient's *Status* field in the hospital database to *RE-NEW*.

The Admin Menu

Admin -> User Roles

Displays the User Roles administration dialog. This dialog allows you to change a user's application roles. The dialog list out all SQL user accounts in the hospital database along with the available roles. The addition of new users to this list must be performed by your database administration team as there is no way of doing this via the tool.

You simply click on the checkbox with the appropriate role and hit the save button. Note that user roles inherit from their sub-roles so in the example below, oa_user has all the attributes of HATUser through to HATAdmin. It is not necessary to select all the roles in between.

NB: Note that you must be a member of the HATSecurity user role in order to access this dialog.

Admin -> Editable Attributes

Displays the Editable Attributes administration dialog. This dialog allows you to define which attributes of DataObjects of a particular type are editable and by which user role. For example, suppose we have a DataObject that represents an "Order" with "Bid" price, Sell" price, "Strike" price then according to the matrix below, for DataObjects of type "Order", HATManagers can edit the "Strike" price attribute and HATControllers can edit all three (user roles inherit). Note that you must define each attribute for each type in order for users of a particular role to edit the details (ie. for DataObjects of type MyOrder which have the same structure as Orders, we would have to define three more rows describing who can edit the attributes). If an attribute is not defined in this matrix then everyone will have read-only access to it.

The Help Menu

Help -> About

Displays details about the HAT.

The Patient List

This panel displays the results of loading in the patients from the hospital. Currently, patients are listed in the datetime order that they were admitted to the hospital. User definable ordering will be added once the delete all patients "feature" is sorted out. When you select a patient from this list the Patient Details and Patient Payload panels are automatically populated with the appropriate data.

When moving from patient to patient the application will check to see if there was any unsaved modifications to the previous patient's payload and prompts you to save them if necessary.

The Main Panel

The main section of the GUI is made up of three panels; the Patient List, the Patient Details and the Patient Payload. The two latter panels are context sensitive to whichever patient is currently selected on the Patient List.

The Patient Details

This panel displays the details of the patient selected in the Patient List. All the details here are read-only and cannot be modified. The most important field is the Rejection Reason

Pop-up Menus

All of the panels that make up the application have context sensitive pop-up menus associated with them. To activate them, you right-click on the appropriate panel.

The Properties File

The configuration of all adjustable elements are stored in a single properties file loaded by HAT at *startup* time. HAT will locate the file "hat.props" in the classpath. A common mistake is to have two properties files available due to a large classpath.

NB: any property that is not defined in this file will have a default values applied from *org.openadaptor.hospital. HATConstants*

Property Details

HAT.logo

The application icon/logo. This is used in the various GUI frames and message boxes.

default: org/openadaptor/hospital/images/hat.gif

HAT.dbRowLimit

The maximum number of patients to read from the database in any one go

default: 100

HAT.dbSlowLoadLimit

if we have requested asynchronous database reads then this number indicates the batch size to use. Possible values are:

- -1: all patient are slow loaded
- 0: all patients are fast loaded
- n: the leading <n> messages slow loaded, all others fast loaded

default: 30

HAT.hospitalName.x

we can define multiple hospitals that HAT can administer. Each one is identified by an incremental number (x) at the end of the HAT.hospitalName attribute. The value for this attribute must be a unique name. This property is required.

HAT.dbDriver.[hospital name]	The driver string used when creating a connection to the database. You check the documentation appropriate to use with your selected driver. The [hospital name] portion must be the same as the one defined in the HAT.hospitalName.x property. Can be omitted but the user will have to manually supply this property in the Hospital Chooser dialogue box.
HAT.dbURL.[hospital name]	The connection URL is specific to the driver you are using so check the appropriate documentation for your driver. Can be omitted but the user will have to manually supply this property in the Hospital Chooser dialogue box.
HAT.dbUser.[hospital name]	The SQL username to use when creating the database connection. Can be omitted but the user will have to manually supply this property in the Hospital Chooser dialogue box.
HAT.dbPassword. [hospital name]	The password to use when creating the database connection. Can be omitted but the user will have to manually supply this property in the Hospital Chooser dialogue box.
HAT.dbHospital. [hospital name]	The name of the hospital table in the database. Can be omitted but the user will have to manually supply this property in the Hospital Chooser dialogue box.
HAT.authorisation-Method	The authentication method to use when authenticating the user. There are two options, "database" or "ldap". default: database
HAT.plugIn	Allows you to load the class objects listed. The plugins must implement the HATPluginIF. The plugins "appear" under the "plugins" menu option. You can specify multiple plugins by using a comma separated list.
[DO type]Validator	Defines the class to instantiate when validating a specific DataObject type. For example, if you have a patient with a payload containing "Order" types then you would need an "OrderValidator" property. Can be omitted.

HAT.fileName

Instead of using a database to store the patients you can use a simple file*. The HAT will provide a read-only view of the patient data contained in a file. It uses the *org.openadaptor.adaptor.standard.FileSource* component to read and interpret the patient details so any properties specific to this component can also be used. Note that the format for these proeprties is slightly different than those for ordinary HAT properties: HAT.<hospital_name>.<property> (eg. HAT.File_A.DOStringReader)

* If you use this option then the database specific properties are ignored.

Here is a sample properties file:

```
HAT.logo = /tmp/HAT.gif

HAT.dbRowLimit = 100
HAT.dbSlowLoadLimit = 30

# define a connection to the MS-SQL hospital "oaHospital"
on myserver.myorg.com
HAT.hospitalName.1 = Hospital_A
HAT.dbDriver.Hospital_A = com.inet.tds.TdsDriver
HAT.dbURL.Hospital_A = jdbc:inetdae:myserver.myorg.
com:1434
HAT.dbUser.Hospital_A = oaUser
HAT.dbPassword.Hospital_A = oaPassword
HAT.dbHospital.Hospital_A = oaHospital

# define file settings
HAT.hospitalName.2 = File_A
HAT.fileName.File_A = /tmp/hospital.dat

# we are using database security tables
HAT.authorisationMethod = database

# we have two plugins
HAT.plugIn = org.openadaptor.hospital.plugins.dummy1,
org.openadaptor.hospital.plugins.dummy2
```

```
# define the validators for known DataObject payloads
OrderValidator = org.myorg.validators.OrderValidator
TradeValidator = org.myorg.validators.TradeValidator
```

The Patient Payload

This panel displays the DataObject payload of the patient selected in the Patient List. It consists of list of the DataObjects that make up the patient's payload and a table to display each of the attributes that make an individual DataObject. Attributes have three elements; the name, the values and the type of the value. Selecting a DataObject will automatically update the attribute table.

To add a new DataObject to the payload, simply right-click on the list and select the appropriate option from the resulting pop-up menu. Similarly, use the pop-up menu to delete a DataObject.

As with the DataObjects, you can add or delete an attribute via the pop-up menus. To edit an attribute you double-click on the attribute element you wish to modify.

NB: there are two ways to save any modifications to the payload; the first is to select another patient and the application will prompt you to save the changes and the second is to use the Save Payload option from the pop-up menu.

Attribute Types: DataObjects can contain data of two attribute types; primitive and complex. Primitive data type possible are:

> String, Int32, Int64, Double, Date, DateTime, Float, Boolean, BigInt and BigFloat.

For a detailed description of this primitive data types refer to the appropriate openadaptor™ documentation.

Complex attributes are those that are formed of an array of business objects which can contain one or more DataObjects of the same type. The value of these attributes is marked as "<ObjectReference>" in the Payload Panel. Clicking on these attributes will cause a subsequent Payload Panel to be opened containing the details of the complex attribute.

The names of the attributes that can be edited are displayed in bold. Double-clicking on the individual columns that make up the attribute allow you to modify that element. Either press the *return* key or click elsewhere in the attribute table to finish editing.

Payload Validation

The HAT is able to validate patient's payloads prior to discharging them. To do this, the *org.openadaptor.hospital.helpers.HATValidator* interface is supplied. This is very simple and defines two methods:

```
public boolean isValid(SimpleDataObject sdo);
public String getMessage();
```

Validators must be provided by the users as each one is applied to a user-specific business object (DataObject). Use the properties file to declare which class is required to validate which business object. The HAT takes the object name (e.g. "Order") and appends the fixed word "Validator" to get the property name ("OrderValidator"). This name is then used to get the full qualified class name from the properties file.

After HAT has instantiated the Validator class it uses the *isValid()* method to check if either the object passed is ok or not. Every validation should generate a qualified text message which can be accessed by HAT after the validation by the *getMessage()* method to inform the user if there is any error or not.

NB: if the user attempts to validate a business object that does not have an associated Validator class then they will get an error message but they will still be able to discharge the patient from the hospital.

Here is a very simple example of a validator that always returns true when the isValid() method is called.

```
package org.openadaptor.hospital.helpers;
import org.openadaptor.dataobjects.SimpleDataObject;
public class myValidator implements HATValidator
{
   public boolean isValid(SimpleDataObject sdo)
   {
      return true;
   }
   public String getMessage()
   {
      return "all ok";
   }
}
```

The Hospital

As HAT is coming up it loads patients from a database source called "hospital". The hospital is a single database table ("DBusMH_Patient") which has been installed to collect Adaptor rejected messages. The pipe component *org.openadaptor.adaptor.hospital.HospitalPipe* is provide to do just this. Normally it passes on messages untouched but catches PipelineExceptions from downstream components. If the Exception type is HOSPITAL then it creates a Patient DataObject (A wrapper around the array of DataObjects).

Every message is an array which contains one or more DataObjects. These objects represent business objects with attributes which contain the business data information.

All hospital entries ("patients") consist of a timestamp and the business data itself. The timestamp indicates the time the patient has been created. Here are the database columns needed/expected by the HAT in a hospital table:

— PatientID
— PatientStatus
— DestAppName
— Subject
— RejectReason
— SourceAppName
— Admitted
— Patient

NB: There are SQL scripts provided under *org.openadaptor.sql* that will create the necessary hospital table and stored procedures.

Multiple RDBMS vendor support

The HAT uses the standard JDBC classes and therefore can connect to hospitals located on databases provided by many different vendors. In order for the HAT to provide support for multiple database vendors, access to the hospitals is controlled via stored procedures. There are reference implementation scripts for MS-SQL and Sybase databases located under the *org.openadaptor.sql* directory to create the database tables and stored procedures.

Known issues: As the HAT currently uses a timestamp range to delete multiple patients from the hospital, it is necessary to order the results by the Admitted datetime field. This will be changed going forward.

The following stored procedures are required:

DBusMH_UpdatePatient	Modifies patient details

	@patientID : the ID of the patient to modify @status : the new status (eg. DISCHARGE_WAIT, PENDING, ...) @payload : the DOXML representation of the patient DataObject
DBusMH_DeletePatient	Deletes a patient from the hospital. Patients are identified by the timestamp when they were admitted to the hospital. If you supply a time range then all patient who were admitted to the hospital between these dates will be deleted. @tsStart : the starting point for the time range @tsEnd : the ending point for the time range @timeAdmitted : the timestamp when the patient was admittedNB: you should pass either the timestamp or the time range.
DBusMH_GetPatient	Returns all the details for a particular patient. @timeAdmitted : the timestamp when the patient was admitted
DBusMH_IsInUserRole	Returns a positive number if the supplied user is a member of the supplied application role, or 0 if not. @roleName : the name of the application role to check (eg. HATManager) @userName : the SQL account of the user you want to check
DBusMH_GetEditableAtts	Returns a list of editable attributes for a given application role and DataObject type @doType : the type of the DataObject (eg. "Order") @userRole : the user role to check against (eg. "HATManager")
DBusMH_UpdEditableAtts	Creates a relationship between a user role and an attribute of a DataObject of a particular type. For example, the "Bid" price attribute of an "Order" DataObject is editable by HATManagers. @doType : the DataObject type

	@userRole : the user role @attribute : the name of the attribute
DBusMH_GETDBUsers	Returns a list of the SQL accounts with access to the hospital database
DBusMH_DeleteUser	Deletes an entry from the DBusMH_User table. Note that this does not effect the ability of the user to access the database, just their roles inside the HAt tool. To delete a user from the database you need to contact your database administration team. @username : the username of the account to delete
DBusMH_UpdUserRole	Creates a relationship between a user account and an application role. @userName : the user account @isUser : equals 1 if the user is a member of the HATUser role @isManager: equals 1 if the user is a member of the HATManager role @isController: equals 1 if the user is a member of the HATController role @isAdmin: equals 1 if the user is a member of the HATAdmin role @isSecurity: equals 1 if the user is a member of the HATSecurity role

3.01 Purpose

The purpose of this chapter is to outline policies and procedures relating to the establishment and administration of training programs for hospital administration residents funded under HARP.

3.02 Policy

(a) HARP supplements the didactic component of accredited graduate programs in health services administration by providing a structured experience within the VA system. Practical experience is from 6 months to 1 year typically after the completion of academic studies. The residency must be a part of the degree requirement.

(b) In addition to HARP, there are a number of other programs in hospital administration and an increasing number of students involved in these programs at the college and university level. VHS&RA encourages health care facilities to seek affiliations (see pt. I, ch. 2) and participate in these programs to increase the number of candidates qualified for appointment to administrative positions in the VA.

3.03 Definition

Hospital administration residents are graduate students pursuing a master's degree in an accredited program of health care administration.

3.04 Establishment

The Office of Academic Affairs (145C) administers HARP activities. Program information, including applicable forms and reporting requirements, is contained in TP 10-27.

3.05 Administrative Producers

(a) See MP-5, part I, chapter 308.

(b) PAID processing requirements are contained in MP-6, part V, supplement No. 1.5.

3.06 Employment Following Completion of Training

(a) Concerned management officials should work closely with the Personnel Officer to ensure that participants are furnished information concerning employment opportunities in the VA after training.

(b) If the resident is not going to be retained at the training site, the resident's completed SF 171 may be forwarded to the Management Support Office (10A5) for referral.

HOSPITAL REGISTRATION AND REPORTING REQUIREMENTS

Every hospital, public or private, shall, by the first of March of each year, register with and report to the department of health the following information for the previous calendar year in a manner prescribed by the director:

(A) Information needed to identify and classify the hospital, include the following:

1. Hospital identifying information, including name, address, mailing address if different than address, county, telephone number, e-mail address, hospital number assigned by the department, and corporate name, if different than hospital name;
2. Name and title of president/chief executive officer;
3. Name, title, and telephone number of individual responsible for submitting hospital registration information to the department;
4. Accreditation/certification status;
5. Name, address, county, and zip code of satellite units;
6. Type of entity that controls operation of the hospital, such as not-for-profit, for profit, government, or other;
7. Name of multi-hospital system of which the hospital is a part, if applicable; and
8. Primary hospital classification from one of the following categories:
   - (a) General hospital; or
   - (b) Special hospital, including:
     - (i) Alcohol and drug hospital;

(ii) Burn care hospital;

(iii) Children's hospital;

(iv) Long term acute care hospital;

(v) Maternity hospital;

(vi) Physical rehabilitation hospital;

(vii) Psychiatric hospital; or

(viii) Other special hospital.

(B) Information on the type and volume of services provided by the hospital, including but not limited to the following:

1. Number of inpatient surgical cases;
2. Number of outpatient surgical cases;
3. Number of surgical operating rooms in the following categories;

(a) Inpatient;

(b) Outpatient; and

(c) Dual purpose (inpatient and outpatient);

4. Number of patients treated in the emergency room and released;
5. Number of patients treated in the emergency room who were admitted to the hospital;
6. Level designation, if institution is a trauma center verified by the American college of surgeons; and
7. Level designation, if institution is a pediatric trauma center verified by the American college of surgeons

(C) Information on the type and volume of services provided by the satellite units, including the following:

1. Types of services provided; and

2. Total number of patients treated (on an outpatient basis) for each type of service provided.

(D) The total number of beds listed by category of inpatient care provided. Report number of admissions (including individuals transferred from another unit within the hospital), number of patient days of care, and number of beds in use for each category of care listed in this paragraph. Beds shall be reported in the following categories:

1. Alcohol or drug abuse rehabilitation;
2. Burn care;
3. Hospice;
4. Level I newborn care service nursery (Level I nursery care beds established in Chapter 3701-84 of the Administrative Code);
5. Level II newborn care service intermediate care nursery (Level II intermediate care nursery beds established in Chapter 3701-84 of the Administrative Code);
6. Level III newborn care service intensive care nursery (Level III neonatal intensive care unit beds established in Chapter 3701-84 of the Administrative Code);
7. Level I obstetric care service (Level I obstetric care service beds established in Chapter 3701-84 of the Administrative Code);
8. Level II obstetric care service (Level II obstetric care service beds established in Chapter 3701-84 of the Administrative Code);
9. Level III obstetric care service (Level III obstetric care service beds established in Chapter 3701-84 of the Administrative Code;

10. Long term acute care;
11. Long term, reported in the following categories;
    (a) Skilled nursing facility beds certified under Title XVIII of the Social Security Act, 49 Stat. 620 (1935), 42 U.S.C. 301, as amended and licensed under Chapter 3721. of the Revised Code, excluding beds reported in paragraph (D)(18) of this rule;
    (b) Nursing facility beds certified under Title XIX of the Social Security Act, 49 Stat. 620 (1935), 42 U.S.C. 301, as amended and licensed under Chapter 3721. of the Revised Code;
    (c) Nursing facility beds certified under Title XVIII of the Social Security Act, 49 Stat. 620 (1935), 42 U.S.C. 301, as amended and Title XIX of the Social Security Act, 49 Stat. 620 (1935), 42 U.S.C. 301, as amended and licensed under Chapter 3721. of the Revised Code;
    (d) Skilled nursing facility beds certified under Title XVIII of the Social Security Act, 49 Stat. 620 (1935), 42 U.S.C. 301, as amended and which are not licensed under Chapter 3721. of the Revised Code;
    (e) Nursing facility beds certified under Title XIX of the Social Security Act, 49 Stat. 620 (1935), 42 U.S.C. 301, as amended and which are not licensed under Chapter 3721. of the Revised Code;
    (f) Nursing facility beds certified under Title XVIII of the Social Security Act, 49 Stat. 620 (1935), 42 U.S.C. 301, as amended and Title XIX of the Social Security Act, 49 Stat. 620 (1935), 42 U.S.C. 301, as amended and which are not licensed under Chapter 3721. of the Revised Code; or
    (g) Long term care beds.

12. Medical/surgical - General;
13. Pediatric intensive care, (beds in a pediatric intensive care unit as defined in paragraph (BB) of rule 3701-84-01 of the Administrative Code);
14. Pediatric - General (services for patients less than twenty-two years of age are provided);
15. Physical rehabilitation;
16. Psychiatric care;
17. Special care;
18. Special skilled nursing (beds certified as skilled nursing facility beds under Title XVIII of the Social Security Act, 49 Stat. 620 (1935), 42 U.S.C. 301, as amended, for which a certificate of need was granted under division (R)(7)(d) of section 3702.51 of the Revised Code and rule 3701-12-233 of the Administrative Code that were in effect on May 20, 1991); or
19. Swing bed (hospital beds with an average length of stay of thirty days or less than may also be used for long term care as certified under Title XVIII of the Social Security Act, 49 Stat. 620 (1935), 42 U.S.C. 301, as amended).

(E) The number of inpatient discharges for each of the following categories:

1. Discharges to home, without referral to home care or hospice services;
2. Discharges to home, with a referral to home care services;
3. Discharges to home, with a referral to hospice care program;
4. Transfers to inpatient service of a hospice care program;

5. Transfers to other hospitals;
6. Transfers to a home licensed as a nursing home under Chapter 3721. of the Revised Code or a facility certified under Title XVIII of the Social Security Act, 49 Stat. 620 (1935), 42 U.S.C. 301, as amended;
7. Total patients expired in the hospital; and
8. Total patients discharged.

(F) The number of employees, including contract employees, by employee type within each of the hospital service categories listed below. Report the number of employees in each type providing patient care services. Report the number of employees as total number of employees and total full-time equivalents.

1. Physician services including interns, residents, salaried physicians, and contracted physicians;
2. Dental services including dentists and dental residents;
3. Nursing services including registered nurses, certified nurse practitioners, clinical nurse specialists, certified nurse-midwifes, certified registered nurse anesthetists (CRNA), licensed practical nurses, and nursing assistants;
4. Pharmacy services including pharmacists and pharmacy technicians;
5. Clinical laboratory including medical technologists, medical technicians and other licensed or certified laboratory personnel;
6. Dietary services including registered or licensed dietitians and dietetic technicians;
7. Radiological services including technologists,

technicians, and other licensed or certified radiological personnel;

8. Therapeutic services including occupational therapists, physical therapists, physician assistants, respiratory therapists, speech/audiology therapists and medical social workers;
9. Mental health services including psychologists and psychiatric social workers; and
10. All other services to include certified or licensed health professional and technical personnel.

(G) Numbers of medical staff delineated by primary area of specialization and category as follows:

1. Area of specialization:
   (a) Medical: Allergy/immunology, anesthesiology, cardiology, dentistry, dermatology, emergency medicine, family practice, gastroenterology, internal medicine, general practice, hematology, neonatology neurology, nuclear medicine, obstetrics and gynecology, oncology, ophthalmology, otorhinolaryngology, pathology, pediatrics, physical medicine, podiatry, psychiatry, radiology, rheumatology, urology, general medicine rotation program, and any other medical specialty; or
   (b) Surgical: Cardiovascular, colon and rectal, general neurological, orthopedic, plastic, thoracic, surgery rotation program, and any other surgical specialty.
2. Categories:
   (a) Active and associate medical staff;
   (b) Active and associate medical staff who are board certified;

(c) House staff;

(d) House staff who are in training positions approved by the accreditation council of graduate medical education or the American osteopathic association; and

(e) House staff who are in training positions approved by the American dental association.

(H) Country (or state if other than Ohio) of resident of patients at the time of admission, reported in the aggregate.

TEACHING PHYSICIAN REQUIREMENTS

Effective July 1, 1996, the Health Care Financing Administration (HCFA) implemented requirements for the documentation of physician services provided in a teaching setting. The goal of these requirements was to avoid duplicate payments for a physician's services through Medicare Part A and Part B. The information contained in this chapter was abstracted from Section 42, Part 415 of the Code of Federal Regulations and from a letter from the Health Care Financing Administration clarifying some of the regulations.

In a teaching setting, physician services provided to individual patients are considered to be the payment responsibility of your Medicare Part B carrier. Conversely, physician services that are furnished for the general benefit of patients (i.e., supervising and teaching residents); and, therefore, considered to be services to the hospital, are the payment responsibility of Part A.

Practices vary widely among and within teaching hospitals with respect to the degree of physician involvement in the care of patients. In some cases, teaching physicians personally direct residents in furnishing patient care services.

In others, residents assume a greater degree of responsibility for the care patients receive, and the teaching physicians exercise only general control over the residents' activities. The most important consideration in determining whether the services of a teaching physician are eligible to be billed to Medicare is the presence of the teaching physician during the key portion of any service or procedure for which payment is sought. The "physical presence requirement" identifies situations when the teaching physician is sufficiently involved in the service, and at the same time, provides a standard that can be readily documented and verified. *Note: the requirements contained in this chapter do not apply to Medicare Managed Care. The documentation rules of the individual health maintenance organisation should be followed.*

Primary Care Exception

There is one exception to the "physician presence requirement." Under this "primary care exception" Medicare may be billed for reasonable and necessary low to mid-level E/M services when provided by a resident without the presence of a teaching physician if all of the following criteria are met:

1. Services must be provided in a center located in the outpatient department of a hospital or another ambulatory care entity in which the time spent by residents in patient care activities is included in determining Part A payments to the hospital. *Please note: this requirement is not met when the resident is assigned to a physician's office away from the center or makes home visits.*
2. Any resident providing the service without the presence of a teaching physician must have completed more than six months of an approved residency

program. The center is responsible for furnishing this information to the Medicare carrier, upon request.

3. The teaching physician may not direct the care of more than four residents at any given time and must direct care from such proximity as to constitute immediate availability. The teaching physician must:
   - Have no other responsibilities at the time
   - Assume management responsibility for those patients seen by the residents
   - Ensure that the services furnished are appropriate
   - Review with each resident, during or immediately after each visit, the patient's medical history, physical examination, diagnosis, and record of test and therapies
   - Document extent of his or her own participation in the review and direction of the services furnished to each patient
4. The range of services furnished by residents in the center include all of the following:
   - Acute care for undifferentiated problems or chronic care for ongoing conditions (including chronic mental illness);
   - Coordination of care furnished by other physicians and providers;
   - Comprehensive care not limited by organ system, diagnosis or gender.
5. The patients seen must be an identifiable group of individuals who consider the center to be the continuing source of their total health care and in which services are furnished by residents under the medical direction of teaching physicians. Although

the residents must generally follow the same group of patients throughout the course of their residency program, the teaching physicians need not remain the same over any period of time.

The "-GE" modifier should be used to denote services provided under the primary care exception.

This primary care exception applies only to specific low and mid-level evaluation and management codes for both new and established patients. The new patient CPT codes to which the exception applies are 99201, 99202, 99203 and their successor codes. Established patient codes to which the exception applies are CPT codes 99211, 99212, 99213 and their successor codes. The teaching physician must be present for higher level evaluation and management codes and all invasive procedures. For this exception to apply, a center must attest in writing that all of the aforementioned conditions are met for a particular residency program.

If a complex situation arises during a service originally scheduled to be furnished under the primary care exception, the teaching physician may bill for the more complex code by using the "-GC" modifier to indicate that the general teaching physician policy, rather than the primary care exception, applies. This will not affect the teaching physician's ability to bill for E/M services furnished by the other three residents under the primary care exception. The key consideration is the unscheduled nature of the Level 4 or 5 E/M service.

There has been some question about the six-month requirement as it relates to all of the residents under supervision of the teaching physician. Medicare has determined that not all of the residents must meet the six-month requirement. If one (or more) of the four residents supervised is still in his or her first six months of training, then the teaching physician must be physically present for the key portion of the encounter between the patient and that resident. The teaching physician would then use the "-GC" modifier to denote that the general teaching physician policy applied.

The teaching physician's activities in connection with the first-year resident should be the type that would not interfere with his or her ability to provide the level of supervision necessary to bill under the primary care exception for his or her activities in connection with the other three residents' services.

Evaluation and Management Services

With regard to evaluation and management (E/M) services (e.g., visits and consultations), the teaching physician must be present during the portion of the service that determines the level of service billed and must personally document his or her participation in the service in the medical records.

If a teaching physician documents his or her presence and participation in the E/M service, the level of service may be selected based on the extent of history obtained, and/or the examination performed, and/or the complexity of the medical decision making. This specific information should be documented by the teaching physician in his or her personal entry in the medical record and may include references to notes entered by the resident.

If the medical decision making for an individual service is highly complex to an inexperienced resident, but straightforward to the teaching physician, the appropriate level of service to be billed should reflect the involvement of the teaching physician in the service. It is the teaching physician's decision whether he or she should perform hands-on care, in addition to the care furnished by the resident. However, in the case of both hospital inpatient and outpatient E/M services the teaching physician must be present during the key portion of the visit. If the teaching physician believes that a key portion of an entire evaluation and management service cannot be identified, then he or she should be present for the entire service.

Radiology Services

The teaching physician need not be present during the actual performance of a radiologic test (or other diagnostic test). The teaching physician may submit a claim for payment for the interpretation when the film is reviewed with the resident, or if an independent interpretation is performed, as long as the radiologic service provided for the patient is meaningful from the standpoint of affecting the patient's course of treatment and is not merely a routine review of a report for purposes of quality control, authorisation, validation or teaching.

If a resident prepares and signs the interpretation, the teaching physician must indicate that he or she has personally reviewed the image and the resident's interpretation and either agrees with it or edits the findings. The body of the resident's note can say, however, that the teaching physician reviewed the interpretation (referencing agreement or edits of the teaching physician). In this situation, a countersignature is acceptable. *A countersignature alone of the resident's interpretation by the teaching physician is not acceptable documentation.*

If the teaching physician's signature is the only signature on the interpretation, the carrier will assume that the teaching physician actually performed the interpretation.

Pathology Services

If a physician submits a claim for payment for a pathology service requiring interpretation, in the capacity of a teaching physician, the following requirements must be met:

- — The service must be personally furnished for an individual patient by the physician
- — The service must contribute directly to the diagnosis or treatment of the patient
- — The service ordinarily requires the performance and exercise of medical judgment by a physician
- — The service must be requested by the patient's attending physician and
- — The service must result in a written narrative report included in the patient's medical record.

In addition to the aforementioned requirements, a clinical pathology consultation must generally relate to a test result that lies outside the clinically "significant," "normal" or "expected" range in view of the condition of the patient.

MEDICAL CONSULTATION AND EXAMINATION AS PART OF LABORATORY SAFETY PLAN

RSO's – note and delete: This section requires minimal tailoring. PIs must be aware of when an employee is entitled to receive medical attention, and must ensure employees are also aware of the process that will be followed.

Employees Who Work with Hazardous Substances

All employees who work with hazardous substances will have an opportunity to receive medical attention, including any follow-up visits that the examining physician determines to be necessary, under the following circumstances:

Signs or Symptoms of Exposure

Whenever an employee develops signs or symptoms associated with a hazardous substance or organism to which the employee may have been exposed in the laboratory, the employee will be provided an opportunity to receive an appropriate medical examination.

Exposure Monitoring

Where exposure monitoring reveals an exposure level routinely above the action level (or in the absence of an action level, the PEL) for an OSHA regulated substance for which there are exposure monitoring and medical surveillance requirements, medical surveillance will be established for the affected employee as prescribed by the particular standard.

Exposure Incident

Whenever an event takes place in the work area such as a spill, leak, explosion or other occurrence resulting in the likelihood of a hazardous exposure, the affected employee will be provided an opportunity for a medical consultation. Such consultation will be for the purpose of determining the need for a medical examination.

Physical Injury

Whenever an employee is physically hurt or injured on the job, the affected employee will be provided an opportunity for a medical consultation and/or examination. Physical injuries include but ar not limited to cuts, burns, punctures and sprains.

Contact the Chemical Hygiene Officer whenever the need for medical consultation or examination occurs, or when there is uncertainty as to whether any of the above criteria have been met.

Workers' Compensation Procedures and Forms

It is very important that even minor job-related injuries or illness are reported. These statistics help the Department of Environmental Health and Safety track trends that may indicate occupational hazards that need evaluation. To report an illness or injury, go to the Workers' Compensation website. University of Minnesota's Policy for Reporting Workers' Compensation Related Injuries is also available on the web. Both sites provide links to the forms listed below.

This policy explains the procedures and provides the necessary reporting forms. As long as the illness or injury is not life threatening, the supervisor should provide the employee with:

- — a brochure describing Workers' Compensation Information for the University of Minnesota;
- — a completed Employers' Authorisation for Care form; and
- — a Work Status Report for the physician to complete and return to the supervisor.

Within 24 hours, the supervisor should complete:

- — a State of Minnesota First Report of Injury form;
- — a U of MN Employee Incident Report form; and
- — a U of MN Supervisor Incident Investigation Report.

Within 24 hours, supervisors must fax the State form to Sedgwick Claims Management Services at (612) 826-3785, and the U of MN forms to the University of Minnesota's Workers' Compensation Department (612)-627-1855.

Medical Examinations and Consultations

In the event of a life-threatening illness or injury, dial 911 and request an ambulance. Employees with urgent, but non-life-threatening, illnesses or injuries should go to the nearest medical clinic. The University of Minnesota's Occupational Medicine Program is located in Boynton Health Service. If off-hours medical attention is required, the employee should be taken to the emergency room at Fairview University Medical Center's University campus. All medical examinations and consultations will be performed by or under the direct supervision of a licensed physician and will be provided without cost to the employee, without loss of pay and at a reasonable time and place.

Information Provided to Physician

The employee's supervisor or department will collect and transmit the following information to the examining physician:

— The identity of the hazardous substance(s) to which the employee may have been exposed;

— A description of the conditions under which the exposure occurred including quantitative exposure data, if available; and

— A description of the signs and symptoms of exposure that the employee is experiencing, if any.

Information Provided to the University of Minnesota

Supervisors should request that the examining physician provide them with a written report including the following:

— Any recommendation for further medical follow-up;

— The results of the medical examination and any associated tests;

— Any medical condition which may be revealed in the course of the examination which may place the employee at increased risk as a result of exposure to a hazardous chemical found in the workplace; and

— A statement that the employee has been informed by the physician of the results of the consultation or medical examination and any medical condition that may require further examination or treatment.

The written opinion will not reveal specific findings of diagnoses unrelated to occupational exposure.

2

Elements and Dimensions of Hospital Administration and Evaluation System

HOSPITAL STAFF AND THE MEDICAL EXAMINER

Please read carefully the sections of this manual that deal with establishing a hospital death as a Medical Examiner case, deaths in the operating room, and deaths occurring in emergency rooms. All discussion applying to the practicing physician applies equally to attending physicians, and hospital personnel whether pathologists, interns, residents, administrators, nursing supervisors, or social workers. Certain special conditions arise in relation to these people and the Medical Examiner which merit separate consideration.

The Hospital Agent

Each hospital shall have a responsible medical professional (such as the Nursing Supervisor), with whom the Medical Examiner can, at any hour communicate. The procedure to follow in reporting a death to the Medical Examiner's Office is the same for hospitals as for practicing physicians. The designated hospital representative shall make the report by phone to the Medical Examiner's Office (206-731-3232, ext. 1) immediately upon determination of death. Pertinent information regarding the decedents medical history is required to be reported at that time. The hospital representative shall submit promptly the following information to the Medical Examiner:

1. Name and age (if known);
2. Date and time of admission;
3. Time of death;
4. Clinical diagnosis (if made);
5. Place, date, time, and manner of incident or violence (if any);
6. Name and telephone number of attending physician;
7. Any other relevant information;
8. If next of kin has been contacted

This will allow Medical Examiner personnel to decide disposition of each case.

In order to assist the Medical Examiner when a death is taken under jurisdiction and investigation, hospital personnel should use the following guidelines. These guidelines are designed to aid in establishing cause and manner of death.

1. Do not clean the body or clothing after death.
2. Special care should be used in cutting and handling of clothing so that valuable evidence such as bullet holes remain intact.
3. All clothing of the deceased should accompany the body.
4. Any IV lines, tubes, catheters, endotracheal tubes, dressings, splints, clamps, and orthopedic devices should be left in place. Therapeutic articles will be returned to the hospital upon request.

5. Any needle puncture wounds to the deceased, made by hospital personnel should be circled in pen and the initials "RX" written next to the circle.
6. Any blood, urine, gastric material, or any body fluid collected at the time of admission should be saved and accompany the body.
7. Admitting blood and urine should be saved on all patients classified in critical condition if their death would result in jurisdiction by the Medical Examiner. This is helpful in detecting concealed homicides.
8. It is permissible for the family to view the body before removal to the Medical Examiner's Office, provided the body is not cleaned or otherwise disturbed. In cases where there is potential criminal, investigation, (e.g., homicidal deaths), viewing should not be permitted and such requests should be referred to the Medical Examiner.
9. Notification of the death to the family should be communicated to the Medical Examiner investigators when they arrive to remove the body. Thus, notification efforts can be initiated and/or coordinated, and not duplicated. The attending physician will be asked to complete a confidential form entitled "Physician's Summary Report". This form seeks information on location of injuries, bullets or other foreign objects, surgical procedures, laboratory and x-ray data, etc. This form is exceedingly helpful in differentiating those marks on the body that are wounds of violence from those that are the result of treatment, e.g., cases with multiple stab wounds. Hospitals will be supplied with a quantity of these forms so that they are readily available. This form must accompany the body to the Medical Examiner's

Office. Cooperation with these procedures is both necessary and appreciated.

After Medical Examiner's investigators receive notification of a death, they are dispatched to take jurisdiction, investigate and transport the body to the KCMEO. A minimum of one investigator is available 24 hours per day. Occasionally, due to multiple calls in rapid succession, an investigator will not be immediately available to respond to the hospital. The person making notification of death should ask if a delay is anticipated. Residential deaths take priority over hospital deaths. This is because hospitals have the staff to care for a body, which is often not possible at a residence.

Medical Examiner investigators will, upon request by hospital personnel, delay their response for up to an hour. Hospital personnel should also inform family members that the Medical Examiner's Office would be contacting them for information necessary for death certification. To this end, whenever possible, hospital personnel should ask responsible family member to remain at the hospital until arrival of Medical Examiner investigators.

Hospital Autopsy

Under no circumstances should the hospital staff request autopsy permission from the family when the death is clearly within Medical Examiner's jurisdiction.

When requested to perform an autopsy by members of the hospital staff, the hospital pathologists should ensure, from the review of the medical history, that the death does not fall under the Medical Examiner's jurisdiction. If, during the course of an autopsy, it becomes clear that the case should have properly been in the Medical Examiner's jurisdiction, the autopsy shall stop. The Medical Examiner's

Office must be consulted to ascertain further direction and guidance. The Medical Examiner is authorized to perform autopsies by RCW 68.50 and King County Ordinance #2878. No permission is needed by the Medical Examiner in order to perform autopsies.

If an autopsy is clearly required for statutory purposes, it will be performed by the Medical Examiner and the physician will be denied the request to seek autopsy permission. Interested attending physicians may request to attend a Medical Examiner's autopsy and/or receive a copy of the autopsy diagnosis and opinion. Release of this information is restricted.

Except in those few instances when there is genuine error, asking the family for autopsy permission is tacit recognition that the death is not in the Medical Examiner's jurisdiction. If it is later decided that it is a Medical Examiner case and the family has refused autopsy permission, this will create needless difficulties.

Instances may arise where the Medical Examiner has jurisdiction in a death, (e.g., hospitalized patient with a fractured femur sustained in a fall at home), but clinicians desire an autopsy authorized by the next of kin to be performed by the hospital pathologist. This can be accomplished only if the following procedure is followed:

1. Notify the Medical Examiner's Office of the death immediately with a clear statement of events, which caused the injury.
2. Inform the investigator taking the call that an autopsy is desired at the hospital for clinical interest. Do not request autopsy permission from the family until assessment has been made by the Medical Examiner that a hospital autopsy can be performed.

3. If the death has been assessed by the Medical Examiner and approval given to seek autopsy permission from the surviving next of kin, the physician can then proceed. A medical examiner case number will be assigned.

Once an autopsy is completed, a copy of the report will be forwarded to the Medical Examiner's Office to complete the record. Similarly, a copy of the death certificate with the identifying KCME case number should be submitted to the Medical Examiner's Office for file. If all prior steps are completed but the surviving next of kin denies autopsy permission, an autopsy may not be authorized by the Medical Examiner over the objections of the family. In some cases, a clinician may wish to perform an autopsy in a case where the deceased has no known next of kin. The Medical Examiner has the authority to authorize autopsies under such circumstances according to RCW 68.50.010 and RCW 68.50.101. If the Medical Examiner agrees to give autopsy authorisation, the physician must sign a Medical Examiner Autopsy Authorisation form agreeing to certain conditions.

SIDS Deaths

Beginning in 1984, there has been a change in the handling and processing of SIDS deaths. Before 1994, infants who were suspected of dying of SIDS were routinely released to Children's Hospital and Medical Center for autopsy. Since 1994, all sudden deaths in infancy are now routinely investigated and examined by the Medical Examiner. This includes scene investigation and recreation, family history, family interviews, routine radiology, autopsy (including histology), and toxicological analysis of body fluids.

Every effort is made by a Medical Examiner Investigator to visit the scene where the death occurred. Additionally, a standard SIDS Scene and Circumstance Protocol is completed on each death so that there is maximum collection of information surrounding these deaths.

After the autopsy examination is completed, and the cause of death is determined to be SIDS, the King County Department of Public Health is contacted so a visiting nurse can have an opportunity for a follow-up visit with the family. At that time, information regarding the local SIDS support group is provided and access to counseling for the families of SIDS's death is made available. Additionally when a death involves an infant or child under the age of 18, the Washington State Department of Social and Health Services is immediately contacted to assess whether or not the individual or family of the child has ever had a Child Protective Service, Family Reconciliation Service, or Child Welfare Service referral. This information becomes an essential part of the investigative report. If the infant or child has had contact with CPS, than a closing case conference is held on a quarterly basis. This interagency agreement is designed to share information on infants and children who come under the jurisdiction of the Medical Examiner and who likewise have had referral to CPS.

Property Disposition

1. Next of Kin is Known

Under no circumstances should the hospital staff take it upon themselves to notify any hotel operator, apartment, or rooming house owner, of the hospital death of any tenant. So doing may lead to the property of the deceased being disturbed, misplaced, or lost to the rightful heirs. If on admission to the hospital, the patient listed the next of kin, he or she may be notified and will likely take charge of property.

2. Next of Kin is Not Known

In cases where no next of kin or legal representative is

known or indicated, the hospital staff or representative should make every effort to locate any next of kin. If after due diligence by the hospital staff or representative, and no next of kin can be located, the Medical Examiner should be notified. Any attempts by the hospital to locate next of kin should be documented and presented to the Medical Examiner Investigator. The Medical Examiner's Office will assume jurisdiction of the death, dispatch investigative staff to the residence, and in the presence of witnesses, take charge of property or the residence, search for next of kin, and arrange for burial as required. Adherence to the above procedure assures that a properly authorized person, in the presence of witnesses, will be the first to enter and search the premises of the deceased.

PRACTICES TO IMPROVE HANDWASHING COMPLIANCE

Hospital-acquired infections exact a tremendous toll, resulting in increased morbidity and mortality, and increased healthcare costs. Since most hospital-acquired pathogens are transmitted from patient to patient via the hands of healthcare workers, handwashing is the simplest and most effective, proven method to reduce the incidence of nosocomial infections. Indeed, over 150 years ago, Ignaz Semmelweis demonstrated that infection-related mortality could be reduced when healthcare personnel washed their hands. A recent review summarized the 7 studies published between 1977 and 1995 that examined the relationship between hand hygiene and nosocomial infections.

Most of the reports analysed in this study reveal a temporal relation between improved hand hygiene and reduced infection rates. Despite this well-established relationship, compliance with handwashing among all types of healthcare workers remains poor. Identifying effective methods to improve the practice of handwashing would greatly enhance the care of patients and result in a significant decrease in hospital-acquired infections.

Practice Description

This chapter focuses on practices that increase compliance with handwashing, rather than the already proven efficacy of handwashing itself. The term "handwashing" defines several actions designed to decrease hand colonisation with transient microbiological flora, achieved either through standard handwashing or hand disinfection. Standard *handwashing* refers to the action of washing hands in water with detergent to remove dirt and loose, transient flora. *Hand disinfection* refers to any action where an antiseptic solution is used to clean the hands (i.e., medicated soap or alcohol). Handwashing with bland soap (without disinfectant) is inferior to handwashing with a disinfecting agent. *Hygienic hand rub* consists of rubbing hands with a small quantity (2-3mL) of a highly effective and fast acting antiseptic agent. Because alcohols have excellent antimicrobial properties and the most rapid action of all antiseptics, they are the preferred agents for hygienic hand rub (also called waterless hand disinfection). Also, alcohols dry very rapidly, allowing for faster hand disinfection.

Given healthcare workers' documented low compliance with recommended handwashing practices, improving compliance represents a more pressing patient safety concern than does the choice of different disinfectants, or attention to other specific issues such as choice of drying method, removal of rings, etc. Of the 14 studies reviewed in this chapter, all study sites utilized hygienic hand rub and/or another method of hand disinfection as standard practice. However, only 2 studies assessed the specific characteristics of handwashing practice (e.g., duration of washing, method of drying) according to established hospital guidelines, while the other 12 studies assessed only whether or not handwashing occurred after patient contact.

Prevalence and Severity of the Target Safety Problem

Nosocomial infections occur in about 7-10% of hospitalized patients and account for approximately 80,000 deaths per year in the United States. Although handwashing has been proven to be the single most effective method to reduce nosocomial infections, compliance with recommended hand hygiene practices is unacceptably low. Indeed, a recent review of 11 studies noted that the level of compliance with basic handwashing ranged from 16% to 81%. Of these 11 studies, only 2 noted compliance levels above 50%. One reason for poor handwashing compliance may be that the importance of this simple protocol for decreasing infections is routinely underestimated by healthcare workers. Recent surveys demonstrate that although most healthcare workers recognize the importance of handwashing in reducing infections, they routinely overestimate their own compliance with this procedure. A survey of approximately 200 healthcare workers noted that 89% recognized handwashing as an important means of preventing infection. Furthermore, 64% believed they washed their hands as often as their peers, and only 2% believed that they washed less often than their peers did.

Opportunities for Impact

Given these findings, opportunities for improvement in current practice are substantial, and efforts to improve current practice would have vast applicability. Many risk factors for non-compliance with hand hygiene guidelines have been identified, including professional category (e.g., physician, nurse, technician), hospital ward, time of day or week, and type and intensity of patient care. These results suggest that interventions could be particularly targeted to certain groups of healthcare workers or to particular locations, to increase the likelihood of compliance. Importantly, this study demonstrates that the individuals with the highest need for hand hygiene (i.e., those with the greatest workloads) were precisely the same group least likely to wash their hands. Finally, another recent study noted that approximately 75% of healthcare workers surveyed reported that rewards or punishments would not improve handwashing, but 80% reported that easy access to sinks and availability of hand washing facilities would lead to increased compliance.

Study Designs

A structured search of the PubMed database (including MEDLINE) and review of the bibliographies of relevant articles identified 14 studies that have examined methods to improve handwashing compliance. Three studies were non-randomized controlled trials (Level 2) that directly compared separate units, or parts of units, in which one area received the intervention and another did not. Eleven studies were before-after studies (Level 3), in which baseline data regarding handwashing rates were obtained during an initial observation period, and then measured again in the time period after a particular intervention. Regardless of the type of study design, details regarding the comparability of the groups under observation were reported in only 4 studies.

Study Outcomes

All of the studies reported changes in percent compliance with handwashing, assessing whether or not handwashing took place. While 13 studies assessed handwashing through observation of healthcare worker behaviour (Level 2), one study assessed soap usage as an indicator of handwashing frequency (Level 3). Two studies also assessed changes in the quality of handwashing. Several studies reported results of surveys conducted following interventions to assess effectiveness and potential adverse events related to the interventions. One study also assessed changes in 2 clinical outcomes (incidence of nosocomial infections and newly detected cases of methicillin-resistant *Staphylococcus aureus*) as a result of interventions (Level 1).

Evidence for Effectiveness of the Practice

Since many different risk factors have been identified for non-compliance with handwashing, it is not surprising that a variety of different interventions have been studied in an effort to improve this practice. While most of the reviewed studies demonstrated significant improvement in handwashing compliance, some did not. No single strategy has consistently been shown to sustain improved compliance with handwashing protocols. In fact, of the studies which assessed longer-term results following intervention, all 3 found that compliance rates decreased from those immediately following the intervention, often approaching pre-intervention levels.

Potential for Harm

While no harm is likely to befall a patient as a result of handwashing, one potential adverse effect of handwashing for healthcare workers is skin irritation. Indeed, skin irritation constitutes an important barrier to appropriate compliance with handwashing guidelines. Soaps and detergents can damage the skin when applied on a regular basis. Alcohol-based preparations are less irritating to the skin, and with the addition of emollients, may be tolerated better. Another potential harm of increasing compliance with handwashing is the amount of time required to do it adequately. Current recommendations for standard handwashing suggest 15-30 seconds of handwashing is necessary for adequate hand hygiene. Given the many times during a nursing shift that handwashing should occur, this is a significant time commitment that could potentially impede the performance of other patient care duties. In fact, lack of time is one of the most common reasons cited for failure to wash hands. Since alcohol-based handrubs require much less time, it has been suggested that they might resolve this concern. In fact, a recent study which modeled compliance time for handwashing as compared with alcoholic rubs, suggested that, given 100% compliance, handwashing would consume 16 hours of nursing time per standard day shift, while alcohol rub would consume only 3 hours.

Costs and Implementation

Interventions designed to improve handwashing may require significant financial and human resources. This is true both for multifaceted educational/feedback initiatives, as well as for interventions that require capital investments in equipment such as more sinks, automated sinks, or new types of hand hygiene products. The costs incurred by such interventions must be balanced against the potential gain derived from reduced numbers of nosocomial infections. Only one study addressed the cost implications of handwashing initiatives. The implementation of a patient education campaign, when compared to the estimated $5000 per episode cost of each nosocomial infection, would result in an annual savings of approximately $57,600 for a 300-bed hospital with 10,000 admissions annually. As others have estimated that the attributable cost of a single nosocomial bloodstream infection is approximately $40,000 per survivor, the potential cost savings of interventions to improve handwashing may be even greater.

Comment

While many studies have investigated a variety of interventions designed to improve compliance with handwashing, the results have been mixed. Even when initial improvements in compliance have been promising, long-term continued compliance has been disappointing. Future studies should focus on more clearly identifying risk factors for non-compliance, and designing interventions geared toward sustainability. Some investigators postulate that better understanding of behaviour theory, and its application to infection control practices, might result in more effectively designed interventions. In addition, any intervention must target reasons for non-compliance at all levels of healthcare (i.e., individual, group, institution) in order to be effective. A more detailed study of the cost (and potentially cost savings) of handwashing initiatives would also foster greater enthusiasm among healthcare institutions to support such initiatives.

ADMINISTRATION OF BLOOD COMPONENTS AND THE MANAGEMENT OF TRANSFUSED PATIENTS

Clinical Governance

In all situations where blood component therapy is given, a quality management system is needed. Quality in the clinical use of blood components implies administering the right amount of the right component in the right way to the right patient at the right time. Quality also includes adequate documentation of both the transfusion process and outcomes. All institutions that transfuse blood products should implement national and local policies and written procedures for:

1. appropriate prescription of transfusion based on clinical guidelines
2. provision of patient information to enable informed consent
3. requests for blood transfusion

4. collection of blood samples for pretransfusion compatibility testing
5. collection of blood components from the hospital blood bank or other storage site
6. storage of blood components
7. delivery of blood components to where the transfusion is to be given
8. administration of blood and blood components
9. documentation of transfusions
10. care and monitoring of transfused patients
11. management and reporting of adverse events
12. staff responsibilities and the training required for these procedures.

It is the responsibility of the prescribing doctor to ensure that blood component therapy is only given when the benefits of the transfusion outweigh the risks; and that the patient is appropriately monitored during the transfusion procedure.

There is an organisational responsibility to ensure that usage of blood is monitored, reviewed and actions are taken to ensure that blood is used safely and appropriately. There should be a clinical/management group, such as a Hospital Transfusion Committee, which reports to the hospital executive and is responsible for the following:

— reviewing transfusion policies and procedures
— reviewing the arrangements for training/continuing education of staff in transfusion policies and procedures
— reviewing adverse transfusion events, including near misses e.g. identified clerical errors
— reviewing the appropriateness of blood transfusion and making recommendations about the proper use of blood and blood components

— recommending corrective action in transfusion practice.

Starting a Hospital Transfusion Committee

Motivation

— Meet with Head of Surgery, Anaesthetics, Haematology, Oncology, Emergency/ICU, O&G, Nursing and Transfusion lab to motivate and recruit members.

— Report a couple of difficult cases to your hospital executive to gain their support. Make them aware of the risk management issues for the institution.

— Set a date and have a clear initial agenda.

— Deal with a topical issue first

— Some States mandate a HTC

Define Role and Terms of Reference

— Always ask: What do you want to achieve?

Primary role of the HTC is usually:

— Provision of an active forum to facilitate communication between those involved with transfusion

— Recommend or perform practice audits

— Monitor transfusion practice compared to institutional, national or international benchmarks

— Provide education to effect change in practice

Membership of the HTC

Institutional Representatives

— Clinicians: Surgery, medicine, paediatrics, haematology, oncology, orthopaedics, O&G, anaesthesia, emergency, ICU

— Executive management

— Clinical risk management/Quality assurance
— Blood Bank scientist in charge
— Nursing
— Other relevant departments e.g. pharmacy

External representatives: ARCBS Transfusion Medicine member. Invited or ad hoc members: Health department

— The initial chair is the most motivated member - You
— Define ongoing Chair at your initial meeting

Activities of the HTC

Goal Setting

— Always have achievable goals
— Break a big problem into smaller components and choose where to start

Agenda Item Suggestions

— Reporting and follow up of adverse reactions to transfusion
— Disseminate and implement national policies and guidelines
— Development and review of institutional transfusion policies and systems eg patient and sample identification
— Identification of staff training requirements in clinical and laboratory transfusion practice
— Development of local educational and training materials as required
— Collection and monitoring of blood ordering practices, use and wastage statistics, errors and incidents
— A great place to start is a small practice audit OR the implementation of general education which will

help raise the profile of the new committee while providing an excellent service for the hospital.

Meeting Frequency

- Frequent enough to get things done, often quarterly
- Pick the best time to suit the majority of members

Other Tips

- Executive commitment and active involvement is important
- Short and informative presentations on topical issues help maintain interest and currency in transfusion practice.
- HTC members have their own networks to assist information exchange - use them.
- Get secretarial support.
- Prompt minutes help.
- Consider providing food - attendance is always better!
- Enjoy it.

Documentation of Transfusions

Good documentation of transfusions allows easy and accurate review of records when required, such as:

- investigation of a transfusion-related adverse event
- performance of quality improvement audits
- management of legal risk.

The following is recommended:

1. The prescribing doctor should document the transfusion decision rationale (based on recognised clinical practice guidelines) in the medical notes. This should detail the outcome of the informed consent process. Patients should be informed of the

potential benefits and risks of transfusion in their particular case and their right to receive or refuse it.

2. The prescription for blood and blood components is the responsibility of a doctor. The prescription should be documented and specify the blood or blood components to be administered, the quantity, the duration of transfusion and any special requirements.
3. A permanent record of the transfusion episode should be kept in the medical notes, including the following:
   - the blood transfusion record (which includes date, number and type of blood component used, donation /batch number, signature of person administering the transfusion and signature of person confirming the identity)
   - the sheets used for the prescription of blood or blood components
   - nursing observations during the transfusion
   - whether or not the transfusion achieved the anticipated benefit
   - management of any adverse events.
4. All records must be held for the required legislated period.

Requests for Blood Transfusion

Completing the blood request form accurately and legibly is an important step in ensuring that the right quantity and type of blood product is made available for the right patient at the right time in the right place. ABO incompatible transfusions are usually due to identification errors.

The following is recommended:

1. Hospitals must have a written policy for blood

transfusion requests, which includes who can prescribe blood.

2. The request form should contain the following information:
   - full patient name
   - unique patient identification number and/or date of birth
   - location of the patient
   - number and type of blood components and blood products requested
   - date and time required, including degree of urgency
   - relevant past obstetric and transfusion history
   - patient's diagnosis
   - indication for transfusion
   - identity and signature of the sample collector and witness.
3. Hospitals must have a policy for the requesting of special blood requirements, such as CMV seronegative, leucodepleted, irradiated etc.

Patient Identification

Correctly identifying the patient, both during collection of the pre-transfusion sample and before starting the transfusion, is vital in avoiding 'wrong blood' episodes.

The following is recommended:

1. Hospitals must have a written policy on the requirements for patient identification.
2. All patients must have a patient identification number and wear an identification wrist band including this number.

3. Patient identity shall be confirmed by asking the patient (if conscious and rational) to state their surname, given name(s) and date of birth and by checking that the identity label is securely fastened to the patient.
4. Where the patient's identity is not known or cannot be accurately confirmed, an alternative reliable method of identification should be substituted and reliably linked to the patient's name once this becomes available.

Notice of the updated identification must be provided to the transfusion laboratory and other relevant departments as soon as possible.

Collection of Blood Samples for Pretransfusion Compatibility Testing

Safe transfusion depends on avoiding incompatibility between the donor's red cells and antibodies in the patient's plasma. The collection of blood samples for pretransfusion compatibility testing must be in accordance with local standard operating procedures7.

The following is recommended:

1. Hospitals must have a policy on pretransfusion sample collection which includes who can collect samples for pretransfusion testing.
2. Only one patient should be bled at a time to minimise the risk of error.
3. The sample must be labelled immediately after the blood has been added, before leaving the patient.
4. Sample tubes must not be prelabelled.
5. The sample tubes must be labelled with the following:

— patient's surname, given name in full

— unique patient identification number and/or date of birth
— date and time of collection
— signature or initials of the collector.

6. It is strongly recommended that addressograph labels should not be used, but if used they must comply with all the requirements of the above point.
7. The collector must verify patient identification by signing both the request form and the sample label to this effect.
8. The hospital blood bank must have policies for dealing with inadequately completed request forms, inadequately labelled samples and discrepancies between the information provided on the request form and sample.
9. The hospital blood bank must verify the patient's ABO and Rh(D) group (and antibody screen if available) against previous records for the patient, and any discrepancies should be resolved before blood components are issued.
10. The hospital blood bank must have a policy for documenting telephone requests.
11. If the request form or blood sample identification is incomplete or incorrect, the request for blood grouping or crossmatching should be refused.

Collection of Blood Components and Delivery to the Ward or Operating Theatre

A common cause of transfusion reactions is the transfusion of an incorrect blood component. This is often due to mistakes when collecting blood components from the hospital blood bank or identification of the patient immediately prior to transfusion.

Hospitals must have a written policy for the collection of blood components and their delivery to the clinical area where the transfusion is to be given. The following is recommended:

1. The policy should define which staff are responsible for this procedure.
2. Blood components requiring refrigeration must be stored only in blood storage refrigerators and not in ward or domestic refrigerators.
3. Blood components must only be stored or transported, as appropriate, in boxes designed and validated for this purpose, including the time for which storage is satisfactory.
4. The staff member removing blood components from the storage facility must have documentation containing the patient's identification details and this information should be checked before removing the blood.
5. Withdrawals and returns of blood components should be documented, including the date and time of removal and return (if applicable).
6. Staff in the ward or operating theatre must check that the correct blood component has been delivered.
7. Only one unit of red cells at a time for each patient should be removed from a blood storage refrigerator unless extremely rapid transfusion of large quantities of blood is required.

Administration of Blood Components

Safe transfusion practice requires a final patient identity check to be undertaken at the patient's bedside immediately before commencing the administration of the blood component. This is vital to ensure the right blood is given to the right patient.

The following is recommended:

1. Hospitals must have a written policy for the administration of blood components which should include identification of the staff responsible for different aspects of the procedure.
2. Prior to issue and transfusion, components must be inspected visually. If there is any evidence of haemolysis, clot formation, abnormal coloration or a significant colour change in the blood bag as compared with the tubing segments (for red cell components), pack damage (e.g. cracks or pinholes), tampering or other suggestion that the unit is not suitable for transfusion, it must not be transfused and should be returned to the issuing blood bank or ARCBS for further evaluation.
3. Transfusion shall not commence until the following has been checked and found to be correct by appropriate staff at the patient's bedside:
   - patient's surname, given name, medical record number or date of birth on both the patient's identification band and the laboratory issue label
   - donation or batch number, blood group and component type against the patient blood group, if applicable and the laboratory issue label
   - statement of compatibility, if applicable
   - expiry date of the unit has not been exceeded
   - expiry date of the crossmatch has not been exceeded, if applicable.

Technical Aspects of the Administration of Blood Components

The following is recommended:

1. Components should be mixed thoroughly by inversion before use and then transfused through an intravenous line approved for blood administration and incorporating a standard (170-260 μm) filter to remove clots and aggregates. It is good practice to change giving sets after 3-4 units or every 12hours.
2. The container must only be entered immediately prior to use.
3. No medication or solutions should be added to or infused through the same tubing with blood or components except 0.9% Sodium Chloride, Injection (BP). ABO-compatible plasma or 4% Albumin or other suitable plasma expanders may be used with approval of the patient's physician. Crystalloid and colloid solutions containing calcium (such as Haemaccel or Gelofusine) must never be added to or administered through the same intravenous line as blood or component collected in an anticoagulant containing citrate as they reverse the anticoagulant effect, resulting in clotting.
4. Plasma thawing devices, intravenous fluid pumps, blood warmers and bedside leucodepletion filters should all be used according to the manufacturer's instructions. Their appropriateness and satisfactory validation for use for blood components should be established prior to use. Equipment should be monitored and undergo regular maintenance. Written procedures for the use of the equipment must be available for staff.
5. If warming is required, an appropriate approved and monitored system must be used that does not haemolyse red cells.
6. Thaw frozen blood components using an approved

method such as a controlled waterbath at temperatures between 30 and 37°C or in an approved microwave device. Care must be taken to prevent contamination of entry ports. The use of watertight protective plastic overwraps is recommended. Do not thaw components in a domestic microwave oven or under hot water directly from the tap.

7. Blood components have been prepared by techniques that aid in preserving sterility up to the time of expiration. If the container is opened in a fashion that violates the integrity of the system for any reason, the component expires four hours after opening. Transfusion of each individual unit should be completed prior to component expiry or within four hours, whichever is sooner.

Use of Blood Filters

A brief summary of the major types of blood filters, their purpose and clinical indications. It is important that blood filters are used in accordance with the manufacturers' instructions.

Care and Monitoring of Transfused Patients

Patients receiving transfusions should be monitored for symptoms/signs of the potential complications of transfusion, and any suspected problems dealt with swiftly. The following is recommended:

1. Hospitals must have a written policy for the care and monitoring of patients receiving transfusions of blood and blood components.
2. Vital signs (temperature, pulse and blood pressure) should be measured and recorded, as a minimum, before the start of each unit of blood component, 15 minutes after the start of each unit and at the end of each transfusion episode.

3. Unless otherwise indicated by the patient's clinical condition, the rate should be no greater than 5 mL/ min for blood components for the first 15 minutes of the transfusion. All blood components should be infused within four hours.
4. The patient should be closely observed during this period since some life-threatening reactions may occur after the infusion of only a small volume of incompatible blood. Temperature and pulse should be measured 15 minutes after the start of each unit of blood or blood component.
5. The possibility of a transfusion reaction should be considered in the event of any deterioration in the patient's condition.

The Management and Reporting of Adverse Events

Many of the serious adverse events following transfusion are unpredictable. The following is recommended:

1. Hospitals should have a policy for the management, reporting, recording and reviewing of adverse events following transfusions of blood and blood components.
2. If a transfusion reaction occurs, the transfusion should be discontinued immediately and appropriate therapy initiated. The transfusion should not be restarted without clinical and/or laboratory review.
3. All significant adverse reactions to transfusion, including possible bacterial contamination of a blood component or suspected disease transmission, should be immediately reported to the hospital blood bank and ARCBS and to the State Health Department as required.
4. As part of the investigation of the reaction, consideration should be given to retaining the implicated blood component for further testing.

GERIATRIC EVALUATION AND MANAGEMENT UNITS FOR HOSPITALIZED PATIENTS

Inpatient care of elders with multiple co-morbidities requires close attention to the special needs and geriatric syndromes that arise in this vulnerable population. One strategy to address the risks of hospitalisation is to provide care by a multidisciplinary team in a dedicated geriatric unit, principally *Geriatric Evaluation and Management (GEM) Units.* This model of care, in many ways similar to coordinated stroke units, may improve mortality and other clinically relevant outcomes compared with outcomes achieved on a general medical ward. An alternative strategy, reviewed elsewhere in this Compendium, is the comprehensive geriatric consultation service, analogous to a typical medical consultation team. In a GEM unit, a multidisciplinary team provides comprehensive geriatric assessment, detailed treatment plans, and attention to the rehabilitative needs of older patients. A typical team is composed of a geriatrician, clinical nurse specialist, social worker, and specialists from such fields as occupational and physical therapy, nutrition, pharmacy, audiology, and psychology. GEM units are typically separate hospital wards that have been redesigned to facilitate care of the geriatric patient. Multidisciplinary team rounds and patient-centered team conferences are hallmarks of care on these units, which, in contrast to geriatric consultation services, have direct control over the implementation of team recommendations.

Practice Description

In all the studies reviewed in this chapter, the GEM unit team included a physician experienced in geriatric medicine, skilled geriatric nurses and rehabilitation specialists. (The latter may not have been on site but were accessible). The teams completed multidimensional geriatric assessments, conducted interdisciplinary team rounds, and provided comprehensive discharge planning. Units were physically separate wards that were designed to facilitate geriatric care. *Acute Care of Elders (ACE) Units* incorporatethe GEM unit design with additional enhancements and admit patients with acute illnesses. ACE units often provide improved flooring and lighting, reorienting devices, and other environmental improvements such as common rooms for patient use. For example, in the ACE unit studied by Landefeld and colleagues the GEM unit concept was enhanced by the use of more nurse-initiated protocols and a greater number of environmental and design modifications. Both styles of unit emphasize the early assessment of risk factors for iatrogenic complications and the prevention of functional decline. Studies of both are included in this study.

Prevalence and Severity of the Target Safety Problem

One-third of hospitalized patients are aged 65 years and older. In 1996, although comprising only 13% of the US population they accounted for 38% of the approximately 31 million discharges from non-government, acute care hospitals. Since all hospitalized older patients are potentially at risk, the target population is quite large. Appropriate selection of patients who are at risk for hospital-related complications and who are likely to receive benefit from this practice, however, would decrease this number. The target safety problems are preventable deaths and hospital-related functional decline in older persons. The number of deaths that could be prevented if the practice were to be widely implemented is unknown. On the other hand, since hospital-related functional decline occurs in 25 to 60% of older hospitalized patients, there is substantial opportunity to improve clinical outcomes. Other clinical problems explicitly studied in controlled trials include cognitive status and nursing home placement.

Opportunities for Impact

Data from the American Hospital Association (AHA) indicate that fewer than half of hospitals providing care for the elderly have geriatric acute care units or offer comprehensive geriatric assessment. Researchers in the field believe the number is increasing. The Department of Veterans Affairs reports that in 1997 there were 110 active GEM units, although some concentrate solely on outpatient assessment.

A recent national survey identified at least 15 active ACE units, with average daily censuses ranging from 5 to 25 patients. Depending on the screening and targeting criteria used to identify eligible patients, the potential for impact could be quite large and raises the question of the physical and manpower capacity of these units to meet the apparent demand.

Study Designs

A structured literature search identified a systematic review that included 6 studies (4 randomized controlled trials; one retrospective cohort study with historical controls, and one published abstract of a randomized controlled trial). We also identified 2 randomized controlled trials of ACE units that were published later. All of the cited studies were single center in design. Five of the studies provided sufficient data to evaluate the baseline level of function of enrolled patients.

Study Outcomes

All-cause mortality was reported in each study. For this outcome, most patients were followed 6 or more months after hospitalisation. Other clinically important outcomes measured in some studies were functional status, cognitive status, length of stay, and discharge rates to institutional settings.

Evidence for Effectiveness of the Practice

In some studies mortality during hospitalisation, at 3 months, or at 6 months was reduced in the intervention group but the differences failed to achieve statistical significance. A meta-analysis of 6 studies found the summary odds ratio for 6-month mortality was 0.65 (95% CI: 0.46-0.91), using both published and unpublished data from the included trials. Tests for heterogeneity across studies were reported with p<0.10 for the pooled analyses. Cognitive function, as measured by the Kahn-Goldfarb Mental Status Questionnaire, showed no statistical improvement over the course of one study, nor did 2 other studies demonstrate improvement, using the Mini-Mental State Examination to assess mental status. Two trials of ACE units examined functional status, using the basic activities of daily living (ADL). Landefeld et al reported statistically significant improvements, while Counsell et al found benefit in a composite outcome of ADL improvement and nursing home placement, but not in discharge ADL levels alone. Two other studies also demonstrated statistically improved functional status in the six months after randomisation and at 12 months follow-up.

In individual studies, GEM units were associated with a higher likelihood of home residence, rather than in an institutional setting (skilled nursing facility or nursing home). The meta-analysis by Stuck et al calculated a combined odds ratio that revealed a statistically significant increase in patients discharged from GEM units who were living at home at 6 months (summary odds ratio 1.80, 95% CI: 1.28-2.53) and 12 months (summary odds ratio 1.68, 95% CI: 1.17-2.41) thereafter. ACE unit trials in a community hospital and a university hospital were also both successful in decreasing patient placement in institutional settings and would likely have strengthened the summary estimate if included. Extrapolating their study findings to the US population, Rubenstein and colleagues estimated that approximately 200,000 nursing home admissions per year could be avoided using their geriatric evaluation unit approach. Winograd noted that this multidisciplinary practice would potentially be more effective if target populations were better identified and enrolled using specific criteria.

Potential for Harm

No data suggest that GEM units were associated with harm.

Costs and Implementation

Implementation of the practice requires construction or redesign of hospital ward(s) to create a suitable environment, training or recruiting experienced staff, establishing selection criteria to determine patient eligibility, and implementing a continuous evaluation process to assess clinical and non-clinical outcomes.

A working group has recommended including costs as an important outcome measure in future studies of GEM units. Applegate and colleagues reported in a later analysis of their randomized controlled trial that the increased costs associated with their intervention study were not balanced by savings in subsequent healthcare spending, but if charges were adjusted for days spent at home (versus in long-term care) the charges were similar. Lower direct costs were demonstrated by one intervention study, particularly after adjusting for differences in survival (mean institutional-care costs per year survived, $22,597 for intervention patients vs. $27,826 for control-group patients). The study by Landefeld et al reported mean hospital charges of $10,289 for intervention patients compared with $12,412 for control patients, with similar median charges (p=0.3). Additional costs of about $75,000 attributable to staffing and physical redesign of the unit resulted in a cost of about $230 per patient in the intervention group. Counsell et al, in a recent large randomized trial of an ACE intervention, reported no difference in hospital costs for patients in the intervention group compared with the usual care group ($5640 vs. $5754, respectively; p=0.68). Included in the costs was $28 per hospital day per intervention patient, representing costs of the geriatric nurse specialist, unit medical director, and unit renovations ($300,000).

Comment

Reasonable evidence supports the use of GEM units, despite varying findings across individual studies with respect to their effectiveness at preventing outcomes such as mortality. Nonetheless, mortality appears to be improved after pooling results of smaller trials. There is good evidence that this model of care decreases nursing home placements, which in itself is a noteworthy finding. Furthermore, the intervention costs may not be significantly higher in these specialized units. The generalizability of the practice requires further examination, and the need for multicenter studies, as advocated by a previous consensus group, has thus far not been undertaken.

Limitations of this practice compared with multidisciplinary geriatric consultation teams include limited bed availability in most units, decreased transferability of geriatric practices throughout a hospital, and a larger resource commitment compared with a hospital-wide consultation team. The advantages of the GEM and ACE unit model are direct control over implementation of clinical recommendations, the presence of dedicated geriatric nursing and rehabilitative staff associated with the unit, and the beneficial effects of a ward designed to address older patients' needs. In sum, the practice of a dedicated GEM or ACE unit carries much promise.

TABLE 1

Randomized Controlled Trials of Geriatric Evaluation and Management Units*

Study	*Study Setting*	*Study Design*	*All-Cause Mortality and Other Outcomes*
Stuck, 1993	6 studies (published 1983-1991) in the US, UK, Australia, and Canada, involving 1090 patients (meta-analysis of Refs. 14-19)	Level 1A	6-month mortality: summary odds ratio 0.65 (95% CI: 0.46-0.91) 12-month mortality: summary odds ratio 0.77 (95% CI: 0.56-1.06)
Applegate, 1990	155 patients in a university-affiliated community hospital, 1985-1987	Level 1	6-month mortality: 10% vs. 21% (p=NS) After 6 months: greatest difference p=0.08 by log-rank test Improvement in ADLs: 3 of 8 ADLs better in intervention group (p<0.05)
Counsell, 2000	1531 patients in a community hospital, 1994-1997	Level 1	Inpatient mortality: 3% vs. 4% (p=0.30) Length of stay: no significant difference Long-term placement or decline in ADLs At discharge: 34% vs. 40% (p=0.027) At 12 months: percentages not reported (p=0.022)
Gilchrist, 1998	222 women on an orthopedic-geriatric service in the UK, 1984-1986	Level 1	Inpatient mortality: 4% vs. 10% (p=0.06) 6-month mortality: 14% vs. 18% (p>0.1)
Harris, 1991	267 patients in an Australian hospital, 1985-1986	Level 1	Inpatient mortality: estimated from Figure 1 in paper, 8% vs. 6% (p=NS) 12-month mortality: 23% vs. 29% (p=NS)
Landefeld, 1995	651 patients in a university-affiliated hospital, 1990-1992	Level 1	Inpatient mortality: 7% in both groups (p=NS) 3-month mortality: 14% vs. 13% (p=NS) Improvement in ADLs at discharge: 34% vs. 24% (p=0.009) Discharged to nursing home: 14% vs. 22% (p=0.01)
Powell, 1990	203 patients in two Canadian teaching hospitals, year not stated	Level 1	Mortality: lower in intervention group; timing not stated (p not stated) Transferred to long-term care: fewer in intervention group (p not stated)
Rubenstein, 1984	123 patients in a VA hospital, 1980-1982	Level 1	Inpatient mortality: 14.3% vs. 15.0% (p=NS)

			12-month mortality: 23.8% vs. 48.3% (p<0.005) 12-month improvement in basic functional status: 48.4% vs. 25.4% (p<0.01) 12-month improvement in mental status: 35.6% vs. 22.4% (p=NS)
Teasdale, 1983	124 patients in a VA hospital, 1981-1982	Level 3	Inpatient mortality: 12% vs. 14% (p=NS) 6-month mortality: 28% vs. 35% (p=NS)

* ADL indicates activities of daily living; NS, not statistically significant.

a. Comparisons are reported as intervention group vs. control group.

PROCESS IMPROVEMENTS BOOST PATIENT SATISFACTION AND QUALITY

Over the past several years, Stanford University Hospital has implemented a multi-faceted response to the healthcare economic crisis. In the January 1993 issue, this publication described wide-ranging restructuring initiatives that resulted in substantial reductions in costs, and these efforts are ongoing. As a parallel to those efforts, and their logical outgrowth, we are using process-management strategies to get at the specifics of quality and cost-effectiveness in our patient-care activities.

Like many institutions, we have initiated many quality improvement efforts in the past decade-some more effective and long-lasting than others. Those that were good sparked dramatic service improvements in some parts of the hospital. Others were little more than "big talk" campaigns that roused a lot of emotion among employees, but really did very little to produce the changes we needed. What our older quality efforts have had in common was a lack of breadth and continuity. One programme might develop an idea that would take care of a problem in one specific area, but it didn't fit in anywhere else. We didn't know how to integrate or coordinate these efforts.

To solve this problem we decided to use a process-management approach to coordinate all our quality initiatives around the goal of moving the organisation toward "patient-centered care." Significantly, although Stanford University Hospital has cut $50 million from the budget over the past four years, our patient satisfaction ratings have never been higher. We attribute this accomplishment directly to the TQM and process-management efforts, and specifically to four aspects that changed the way we previously thought of quality management. This process:

— Challenged us to think through the identity of the hospital's "customers," both internal and external.
— Increased the amount of feedback to caregivers on concerns expressed by our patients.
— Forced us to use quantitative measures to control and evaluate the effectiveness of routine sub-processes.
— Kept us accountable and focused on our mission with regularly scheduled review sessions.

With support from top management, a Patient-Centered Care Team (PCCT) brought together managers from all areas of the hospital. Under the direction of our consultants, Shaw Resources, the team decided to limit its work initially to those processes that directly involve patient care, eliminating such behind-the-scenes functions as data processing. We also narrowed our focus to inpatient hospital care; outpatient processes will be tackled at a later date.

The Patient-Centered Care Team then did something that we had never considered before-we "walked through" a typical hospital experience, from admission to discharge, from the patient's point of view. We supplemented our biweekly meetings with outside reading assignments and information gathered in videotaped focus groups with former patients. What our quality efforts had in common was a lack of breadth and continuity. It was a startling experience. The Customer-Supplier Process Model (see chart, page 3) used by Shaw Resources as a template for our work forced us to look at our organisation from a totally new perspective. We began analysing processes through the eyes of the patient, rather than from our own experience or knowledge of what was efficient or cost-effective.

The next step was to identify specific areas to address through separate "process management teams" of the Patient-Centered Care Team. We chose to concentrate in this first phase on the following processes and we launched one team per month until all seven were up and running:

— Admit Patient
— Provide Laboratory Support
— Provide Hotel Services
— Provide Patient/Family Support
— Manage Patient Care
— Provide Diagnostic & Treatment Support
— Management Complaints

A "process owner" was identified for each team (based on who had the most resources and was most accountable for that process) and that individual selected appropriate people to serve. Team members set the agenda and frequency of meetings.

After a team has been in operation for a while, members report back on their work and results to the Patient-Centered Care Team at six-month intervals. The accountability of these "report-back" sessions is integral to the forward movement of each team. In addition, these report sessions have offered an opportunity for collaborative problem solving by top administrators. Any early fears we had about team members becoming too focused on boxes and circles of a process flow-chart were dismantled when the report-back sessions started. The Patient-Centered Care Team keeps its focus on the big picture and the individual teams concentrate on the details of measurement, change, and improvement.

All of the teams have experienced "breakthrough" insights in identifying customers and customer expectations, and using measurements that quantify change. Described here are examples from the Manage Patient Care Team and the Provide Diagnostic & Treatment Support Team.

Understanding Patient Expectations

"Patients have high expectations when they come to Stanford University Hospital," comments Joann Zimmerman, assistant director of nursing for medical/surgical. "They expect expert care and take for granted the technology or experimental drugs that might save their lives. But if their meal is left on a table just outside their reach from the bed, or if it takes ten minutes before someone responds to their call bell, they are highly critical. From our point of view, we were providing quality care. But we quickly learned that patients have different expectations and definitions of 'quality' than we do as healthcare providers." The Manage Patient Care Team is different from all others because its members are homogenous-all are RNs with similar education, professional experience, job responsibilities, problems, and the same manager, Zimmerman, who is also the "process owner" of this team. In many ways, this homogeneity allowed the group to coalesce and move into action quickly.

The Manage Patient Care Team asked nurse managers to proactively collect patient complaints based on defined quality measurements. "This was a difficult transition for many of us," Zimmerman says. "No one wants to hear a complaint and it took a great deal of effort to convince units that there would be no shame attached to having a high number of complaints." In a two-month period, managers of ten general medical-surgical units gathered 178 documented complaints. "We didn't expect that patients would be dissatisfied with nursing care. We were Wrong!" "There were more complaints than we anticipated, and we didn't expect that patients would be dissatisfied with nursing care," Zimmerman says. "We were wrong. The number one complaint was related to nursing care, followed by an uncaring attitude from caregivers, call light response time, and response time to requests for pain medication."

Responding to Complaints

In addition to collecting patient complaints, the members selected as a starting point two processes that are very important to the patients-pain medication delivery time and call button response time. The team discovered that, typically, patients were being supplied with pain medication within 4.5 minutes of their request, but that this respectable number was averaged from a wide range of response times. More study showed that the delay almost universally was caused when no pain medication appeared on orders after surgery. The nurse had to locate the physician and obtain a pain medication protocol before any drug could be obtained or administered. This could be a time-consuming process. As a result of these findings, doctors' orders on all patients admitted to general medical-surgical units are now scanned when the patient arrives to see if a pain medication protocol is indicated. If none is noted, the physician is contacted at this point-before the patient is in pain and requesting medication. Reducing call button response time is a lengthier, more involved challenge. According to our previous research, we knew we answered 95 percent of all call lights within one minute. What we didn't realise was that "answer" had a different definition to us than it did to the patient. We were pleased to be able to say that within 60 seconds, a patient pushing a call light could expect to hear a clerk respond with a reassuring "The nurse will be right with you." But from the patient's point of view, the call light was not "answered" until someone appeared in the room, which could be as much as ten to 15 minutes later.

The team decided that the best way to adapt this process to fit the patients' expectations is to train clerks to categorize call lights (elimination, pain med, comfort, etc.) and then give patients a more realistic time estimate of when their need or request will be met. For example, a patient with a low-priority request in the comfort category will be told "The nurse will be there in five minutes" so that he or she won't be expecting someone to pop in the door within seconds. Soon, the nurses' beepers will be coded so that they know immediately what patients' needs are by category and, therefore, how quickly they need to respond.

"We've always measured our quality by the standards of the healthcare professionals, not by the measures of patients," adds Zimmerman. "It was the caregiver's agenda, not the patient's agenda. Through process management, we got a different viewpoint on what we have taken for granted." Nurse managers now make rounds three to five times per week to interview patients about the quality of care. Constant and consistent communication is nipping off minor annoyances before they have time to bud into major problems, and the patient "inputs" become valued information for the Manage Patient Care Team to study.

Unexpected Results

Meanwhile, members of the Provide Diagnostic & Treatment Support Team were getting acquainted. This group brings together managers of several nursing units and departments that provide diagnostic and treatment services-the cath-angio lab, the cardiology lab, dialysis, endoscopy, nuclear medicine, the pharmacy, the pulmonary/ blood gas lab, the neuro lab, radiation oncology, radiology, rehabilitation services, and respiratory therapy.

I think one reason that our previous quality efforts have not been the solutions we hoped for is that they tried to solve problems within the confines of one department," she adds. "Once we saw the flow-charts it was clear to us that this would not work. Patients move from one area to another and they don't care that they may have crossed an organisational boundary. They judge their total experience in the hospital. This was even more dramatic when we took the additional step of completing a flow-chart from the patient's perspective."

The team has identified numerous areas for further improvement and measurement. Some of these are: (1) patient transport; (2) clarification of physicians' orders; and (3) turnaround time of reports to physicians.

Already, minor process improvements are showing results. Reminder calls to outpatients about their appointments in the cardiology lab have limited late arrivals to one since March of 1993. Routine surveys of patients before and after respiratory therapy treatments sparked a new policy of re-orientation for professional staff that has been gone on leave. "Patients can spot when a caregiver is not at ease working with new equipment," Lanigan explains. "This discomfort is jarring to the patient's expectations of what the treatment experience should be like. By interviewing respiratory therapy patients we discovered this had occurred when someone had been on leave for a while and new equipment had arrived during that period. The respiratory therapy department subsequently changed its process to 'check off' returning staff on familiarity with new equipment or procedures." Simultaneous with the patient-centered care efforts at Stanford was a move to decentralize support services to the point of care. This major organisational change, which was initiated earlier as part of our cost-reduction programme mes, enhanced the work of the process management teams and helped boost our patient satisfaction ratings. For example, studies showed that patient treatments were often delayed while supplies were delivered to the unit. Now the hospital has a mini-supply room on each floor, controlled by a state-of-the-art computerized inventory and tracking system. We can now guarantee that supplies will be available within five minutes.

Support Service Assistants

Another structural shift was the merger of housekeeping and transportation personnel and the decentralisation of these services. Stanford Hospital now has "support service assistants" (SSAs) assigned to each unit to provide housekeeping and transport services. The same employee cleans a patient's room, takes him or her to X-ray, and delivers meals. The contributions to patient-centered care have been enormous:

- It has reduced the number of faces a patient sees in the course of a day. (Too many interactions from too many different people-a high probability at a teaching hospital-are a major source of patient complaints.)
- It personalizes the service patients do receive. It is not "housekeeping" that is making their rooms spotless —it's Rose, or Jose, or Mike.
- It has given the SSAs more feelings of connection and ownership for doing a good job. They see immediately how their jobs affect patient care. Hours

of training, coaching, and preaching about the importance of prompt service cannot equal the impact of seeing for themselves how a patient feels to sit and wait for a wheelchair.

— It has saved money by eliminating a second layer of supervision. SSAs report to the nurse manager in the unit.

The introduction of SSAs and decentralisation has not been without challenges. Nurse managers were unaccustomed to hiring and supervising this level of personnel and needed additional training. Previously, these support employees were distanced from the patients and had little direct contact with them. Now they deliver their services bedside and get to know patients by name and face-and they care about the outcomes. "Before I never thought about why a room was empty. My job was to clean. Now I know that Room 304 is empty because Mrs. Smith has died." SSAs now receive training and counseling on death and dying.

Next Steps

As the process management teams continue their work, the Patient-Centered Care Team is wrestling with how to attack our next set of challenges. We have identified three "next steps":

— Educate staff on the process management methodology, especially the value of complaints in improving patient-centered care. Currently, process management teams involve fewer than 100 of the approximately 4,700 employees of the hospital. Training needs to take a variety of forms and levels of depth to accommodate the diverse range of educational levels, cultural backgrounds, and licensed and non-licensed positions.

— Continue to effectively manage the overwhelming amount of data available to the process management teams. Unlike some organisations, a hospital already has a wealth of information recorded. The challenge is to analyse it productively and feed it back to employees in a way that is meaningful and produces change and improvement.

— Devise reward systems that are valued by our people. In the '90s a reward for a job well done no longer necessarily needs to be money. Many employees prefer a flexible schedule or an extra day off to a bonus in the next paycheck.

— Dovetail patient-centered care activities with process management.

There are no quick fixes in a healthcare organisation-our problems are too complex, our issues too critical to the well being of our patients. But process management has pointed us all in the same direction with the same goal in mind. We are seeing real change and real results that will be long-lasting because they are altering the core infrastructure of our organisation.

"Outstanding performance and patient-centered care are not based on how many resources you have but on the quality of your leadership," says Zimmerman. Process management has taken our leadership skills up a notch and everyone connected with the hospital-physicians, staff, and most of all, patients-is benefiting.

CRITICAL PATHWAYS

Burgeoning concerns regarding patient safety, variable healthcare quality and increasing healthcare costs have led to the introduction of clinical management tools that have their origins outside of the traditional healthcare sector. Primary among these innovations has been the implementation of critical pathways, administrative models that streamline work and production processes. Critical pathways have been utilized extensively in several different business sectors including the construction and automotives industries. It is theorized that the adaptation of pathways to healthcare, particularly inpatient care, may help ensure the delivery of quality care and decrease the occurrence of medical errors.

Practice Description

Although closely related to clinical practice guidelines, pathways more directly target the specific process and sequence of care, frequently plotting out the expected course of an illness or procedure with associated prompts for appropriate interventions. Also known as clinical pathways and care maps, pathways are generally multidisciplinary by design and may incorporate the responsibilities of physicians and nurses with those of ancillary medical providers including pharmacists, physical therapists and social workers. They are regularly intercalated into the point-of-care and may, in some cases, incorporate or even replace traditional chart documentation. In addition, pathways are often evidence-based and may even be integrated with locally or nationally developed clinical practice guidelines. Most pathways, however, are locally developed and are most frequently implemented at the level of the hospital or medical center as part of a cost-containment or quality assurance initiative.

Prevalence and Severity of the Problem/Opportunities for Impact

It is well established that the methods currently used to disseminate medical information are both cumbersome and inefficient. Even medical advances that are well entrenched in the literature and of unquestionable value are not routinely or universally implemented. A study of patients treated for myocardial infarction in Connecticut, for example, revealed only 50% of patients received the most basic beneficial treatments (aspirin and beta-blockers) at the time of admission. A second report suggested that 3500 myocardial infarctions would be averted and 4300 lives would be saved annually if all eligible patients with coronary artery disease were prescribed beta-blockers. Critical pathways, if able to beneficially alter healthcare provider performance and ensure that effective patient safety strategies were practiced on a widespread basis, could be powerful agents in the prevention of medical errors, in addition to any beneficial impact they might have on overall healthcare quality.

Study Design

There is a dearth of well-designed studies analysing the extent to which critical pathways change physician behaviour and patient outcomes. Even fewer relate specifically to the topic of patient safety. There are no systematic reviews of pathways and most of the published work describes the non-randomized implementation of pathways in which it is often difficult to differentiate effects of the pathway from secular trends. The vast majority of these studies describe the implementation of a pathway for a specific surgical procedure and use historical controls with a retrospective before-after study design.

Four randomized controlled trials investigated the impact of the implementation of pathways. There are also several studies with non-randomized concurrent controls with enrollment in the intervention arms being completed at the request of the attending physician. The latter group of studies also included historical control groups. There is one prospective before-after trial in which the control group actually shifted to receive the intervention after a washout period. Finally one study used historical controls and concurrent controls from other hospitals in the region. The salient features of these papers.

Study Outcomes

The great majority of the cited studies reported at least one clinical outcome (Level 1) with the most commonly reported variable being diagnosis-related complications. Very few of the studies reported more definitive endpoints, such as mortality. Most of the included studies reported surrogate clinical end-points (Level 2) as the major study outcome variables, usually length of stay and re-admission rates. The relative utilisation of certain interventions including medications, laboratory tests and radiology studies was also commonly reported. In addition, most of the studies also included an analysis of the changes in costs associated with instituting the pathway. Some of the studied pathways did include other recommendations for interventions germane to the field of patient safety, including the use of indwelling urinary catheters and prophylactic preoperative antibiotics, but these outcomes were rarely reported.

Evidence for Effectiveness of the Practice

Several of the randomized controlled trials provide at least some evidence that critical pathways can be effective in influencing healthcare provider behaviour. One study evaluated the effectiveness of a pathway for the treatment of asthma in children admitted to a non-ICU hospital setting. Those patients treated under the pathway, when compared to the control group undergoing "usual care," had a shorter length of stay as well as decreased hospital charges and medication usage, but no change in complication rates. Although the results are somewhat promising, the study was likely skewed by a significant Hawthorne effect, as patients treated under the pathway were placed on a separate clinical ward than those undergoing usual care (although the same physicians cared for both groups of patients). This study found no impact on the rate of complications, which provides little encouragement regarding the ability of pathways to reduce medical errors and enhance patient safety.

A second randomized trial investigated the utility of a pathway for the treatment of patients undergoing knee and hip replacement at an academic medical center in Australia. Implementation of the pathway was followed by significant decreases in the length of stay and shorter times to patient mobilisation and ambulation. More importantly, it showed a decrease in the incidence of medical complications, including readmission rates (although this change did not reach statistical significance). The study, although fairly small at 163 total patients, represents some of the most convincing evidence that pathways may be effective in decreasing complications.

A third randomized trial, performed by the same Australian group, evaluated the effect of a pathway for the treatment of patients with hip fracture. Implementation of this pathway, which provided recommendations regarding medications, laboratory and radiology testing and discharge planning, resulted in a significantly shorter lengths of stay without any concomitant change in complication rates. The study was rigorously conducted and complication rates were meticulously documented, but no information regarding the effort needed from clinicians to comply with the pathway was presented.

A final trial used cluster randomisation to investigate the effectiveness of a critical pathway for the treatment of community-acquired pneumonia in 19 Canadian hospitals.

The pathway, which was initiated upon presentation of the patient to the emergency department, included recommendations for the use of a specific antibiotic and provided a clinical prediction tool to aid in decisions regarding hospital admission. Following admission, a study nurse also regularly placed guideline-based recommendations in the chart regarding changing to oral antibiotic therapy and discharge planning. The pathway showed impressive results in terms of cost containment, with a shorter length of stay and a smaller percentage of inappropriate admissions. However, there were no significant changes in the clinical parameters measured, including mortality and complication rates. In addition, it is difficult to dissect the effect of the pathway from that of the other elements of the multifaceted intervention.

The second strata of studies were less encouraging. A prospective before-after evaluation of the implementation of a pathway for the administration of supplemental oxygen for hospitalized patients showed the pathway was associated with markedly elevated costs without any significant clinical benefit. This study, which used an intensive 3-tiered strategy including an oxygen order form, the posting of the pathway in patient rooms and a research nurse providing immediate audit and feedback, doubled the cost of providing supplemental oxygen. Although it did change some of the physician prescription practices, this alteration in practice resulted in no appreciable clinical effect.

At least 2 other studies compared an intervention group with a non-randomized concurrent control group (thus introducing the possibility of selection bias) as well as to historical controls. In a study evaluating the impact of a critical pathway on the treatment of patients undergoing neck dissection, the length of stay and total costs were significantly lower for the pathway group when compared with those of the historical controls. However, the differences disappeared when the concurrent control group was used. In the other, a study of a pathway for the treatment of asthma exacerbations, the pathway resulted in improvements in resource utilisation that were significant compared to both historical and concurrent controls. However no changes were noted between the groups in readmission rates or medical outcomes.

Finally, there are a great number of observational before-after studies of pathways, the vast majority of which relate to specific surgical procedures. Few of these studies account for secular trends and their capacity for judging the effectiveness of critical pathways is limited, at best. In addition, a recent evaluation of pathways for patients undergoing a variety of surgical procedures compared the intervention group to both historical controls and to patients from similar hospitals in the same region in an attempt to correct for such secular trends. Although implementation of the pathways resulted in significant decreases in length of stay when compared to the historical controls, these differences disappeared when the pathway groups were compared to the concurrent control groups from the other hospitals. An additional study of the effect of a pathway on the treatment of acute myocardial infarction demonstrated that the improvements seen in the intervention group were likely secondary to secular trends and not an independent effect of the pathway. These powerful results cast a great deal of doubt over those studies that demonstrated effectiveness of the pathways in comparison to historical controls alone.

Potential for Harm

There are theoretical concerns that pathways may result in adverse patient outcomes as a result of shortened length of stay and a dependence on "cookbook medicine," although there is little support for this in the literature.

Although many studies report cost savings associated with instituting pathways, very few detail the costs of developing and implementing them. One report attempted to put a dollar figure on the development of a pathway for the treatment of patients undergoing knee replacement surgery; however the reported estimate ($21,000) did not account for the time staff physicians spent on the project. The expense of developing critical pathways in terms of physician time commitment and actual financial outlay is unknown. In addition, most pathways are developed on the local level and require a great deal of initiative and expertise on the part of the hospital or medical center. Whether most centers have access to these resources is unclear.

Physicians and other providers are also not universally welcoming of critical pathways. They are considered intrusive by some providers and evidence of "cookbook medicine" by others. The developers of pathways must be careful to allow for clinical judgment and flexibility in the pathways or they are likely to be ignored or applied too rigidly.

Comment

There is conflicting evidence regarding the efficacy of critical pathways as a method to modify healthcare provider behaviour and a means of implementing patient safety initiatives. Although a few studies suggest they may impact physician practice and, to a lesser extent, complication rates and other clinical outcomes, the data are inconsistent and more studies are needed. Additionally it is unclear whether the costly development and implementation of pathways represents an appropriate use of limited healthcare resources. Finally, there is very little information on the application of pathways to patient safety.

CONCEPTUAL APPROACH AND FRAMEWORK FOR MONITORING AND EVALUATION

Evaluating HIV/AIDS prevention and care programme mes is a never-ending challenge, but recognizing its importance in improving current interventions may help to enhance the success of future initiatives.

There are probably as many definitions of "programme evaluation" or "evaluation research" as there are programme evaluators. Our approach to evaluating HIV/AIDS prevention and care programme mes is best captured by a description of evaluation provided by Michael Quinn Patton:

> "I use the term evaluation quite broadly to include any effort to increase human effectiveness through systematic data-based inquiry. When one examines and judges accomplishments and effectiveness, one is engaged in evaluation. When this examination of effectiveness is conducted systematically and empirically through careful data collection and thoughtful analysis, one is engaged in evaluation research.... Evaluation is applied research, or a type of "action science." This distinguishes evaluation research from basic academic research....The purpose of applied research and evaluation is to inform action, enhance decision-making, and apply knowledge to solve human and societal problems....Applied evaluative research is judged by its usefulness in making human actions and interventions more effective and by its practical utility to decision makers, policymakers and others who have a stake in efforts to improve the world."

Such an evaluation approach is utilisation-focused. This approach emphasizes the interests of key stakeholders and primary users of the information at all levels, for example the donor, the host country, and the implementing agencies. It applies socio-epidemiological research to identify ways to improve the design and implementation of HIV/AIDS prevention and care programme mes.

This chapter first describes several considerations that are fundamental to planning an evaluation effort. It then presents a comprehensive framework for country programme mes by explaining the major types of evaluation and discussing several important issues related to planning evaluation programme mes and improving their ability to measure programme effects.

Basic Considerations

Several considerations underlie the decisionmaking process about HIV/AIDS programme evaluation. The selection of an appropriate evaluation concept for an AIDS prevention programme is crucial because it determines the guiding philosophy behind the actual evaluation process. A number of theorists and evaluation practitioners have proposed various conceptual approaches to evaluation. These approaches differ in their conception as to what evaluation is, what the relationship with the primary client and other stakeholders should be, who should be making the relevant value judgments regarding the programme , and the criteria for judging the evaluation process itself.

The conceptual approach debate was, and is for the most part, a debate about the best ways to measure and interpret change. It has highlighted a series of methodological dimensions among which there are variations in emphasis. These dimensions focus attention on some of the options available for making decisions about methods. Today, for example, there is consensus that both quantitative and qualitative data are valued and recognized as legitimate for programme evaluation. In fact, these methods are by no means incompatible and should be used in combination.

Deciding what and how much data to gather in an evaluation involves difficult methodological decisions and trade-offs between the quality and utility of information.

An evaluation approach that uses multiple data collection methods, both quantitative and qualitative, is more likely to address diverse evaluation needs than is a more limited approach. At the same time, research priorities must be sensitive to competing needs for resources in an environment in which the HIV/AIDS epidemic is growing rapidly and evaluation is sometimes considered a luxury. It is a major task of the evaluator to match research methods to the reality of particular evaluation questions and to the available resources.

There is also a need for evaluation researchers to play an active role, not merely a consultative one, in making design decisions for programme assessments. Although a programme evaluator should be a neutral scientific observer, he or she can also mediate between different stakeholder groups, can enable others through a participatory evaluation approach, and can advocate for the dissemination of evaluation results within the larger arena of decisionmaking. Planning evaluation and data collection activities in a participatory fashion is essential for achieving the delicate balance between practical needs and methodological desirability. Key stakeholders should be included in the planning process and every effort should be made for effective use of limited resources. Ensuring active support and participation of key stakeholders who have an interest in the results obtained by various data collection systems is particularly important for programme mes funded by external donors that use host country institutions for data collection activities. Data produced by these efforts will have a better chance to be timely and of acceptable quality. Whenever possible, participants, including implementing institutions, host-country collaborators and local representatives of donor agencies, should attempt to reach consensus regarding data needs.

A Comprehensive Evaluation Framework for Country Programme mes

HIV/AIDS prevention and care programme mes need to be evaluated at different phases of the programme cycle. A framework for comprehensive programme evaluation. All stages of evaluation have to be considered together to provide an overall picture of the programme because no single data collection approach can supply all the information necessary to improve programme performance or affect policy change. Multiple complementary evaluation approaches and multiple methodologies (qualitative and quantitative) have to be applied to address different evaluation needs.

Formative Evaluation

Formative evaluation should be conducted during the planning (or replanning) stage of a prevention and care programme to identify and resolve intervention and evaluation issues before the programme is widely implemented. This is the time when flexibility is greatest and programme sponsors are freer to make decisions about how to proceed.

Formative evaluation explores the need for interventions, provides the information necessary to define realistic goals and objectives for the programme interventions, and helps programme planners make tentative decisions about effective, feasible intervention strategies and how to carry them out. Formative evaluation can also be used as an exploratory tool as the project is being carried out to provide feedback to project managers to help them adjust programme objectives to changing situations. Formative evaluation research can identify unacceptable or ineffective intervention approaches, designs, and concepts.

Because of the urgency of the HIV/AIDS problem, many prevention programme mes have rushed to carry out interventions without preparing first by conducting thoughtful formative evaluation. The lack of this type of evaluation is particularly felt in community-based interventions designed to reduce sexual transmission of HIV. In many cases, interventions have been based on ideas developed outside of the context of the lives of the people to whom the interventions have been delivered. The literature on behavioural change interventions is full of examples of ideas that made perfect sense in the abstract but failed completely in the "real world," mainly because the ideas were unacceptable to the target audience or were not stated in ways that were relevant to the lives of those people. A fuller understanding of the issues might well have led planners to redesign the intervention to make it more appealing to the selected audience. Fortunately, this situation is changing because formative evaluation is now being applied more frequently in designing prevention programme mes.

Formative evaluations use a mix of research methods that can rapidly provide relevant information to programme designers. These methods include:

- — reviews of existing information;
- — focus group discussions;
- — individual in-depth interviews;
- — participant observations; and
- — short quantitative surveys with structured questionnaires

The most frequently cited methodological criticism of formative evaluation is its lack of external validity or generalizability. Because the results of the evaluation derive from small-scale rapid assessment procedures and/or pilot studies, one cannot generalize from them to a larger population. Despite this limitation, formative evaluation research can usually identify unacceptable or ineffective intervention approaches, designs, and concepts. However, even with adequate formative evaluation at the programme planning stage, there is no guarantee that a prevention programme will be effective when finally implemented; it may not be implemented adequately enough to be effective.

Process Evaluation

Once activities are underway, there is a need to examine whether they are being carried out correctly, on time, and within budget. Process evaluation addresses such basic questions as,

> "To what extent are planned intervention activities actually realised?" and "What services are provided, to whom, when, how often, for how long, and in what context?" Both input (the basic resources required in terms of manpower, money, material, and time) and output (the immediate service improvement expressed as distributed commodities, trained staff, and service units delivered) are key elements of process evaluation. These questions are often answered in quantitative terms. Qualitative evidence of how and why a prevention programme works or fails to work is equally important in answering process evaluation questions. Process evaluation requires getting close to data, becoming intimately acquainted with the details of the programme , and observing not only anticipated effects but also unanticipated consequences. An understanding of the processes through which intervention activities achieve effects can help to explain the outcome of the intervention. Process evaluation, however, does not demonstrate whether interventions are effective.

Process evaluation can also play an important role in improving or modifying interventions by providing the information necessary to adjust delivery strategies or programme objectives in a changing epidemic. Process-oriented evaluation is carried out throughout the course of the programme implementation and should use different methodological approaches to assess service delivery, ranging from reviews of service records and regular reporting systems, key informant interviews, exit interviews of service users, direct observations by 'mystery clients' (for example, in sexually transmitted infection [STI] and voluntary counseling and testing [VCT] services) to quantitative population-based surveys to assess programme coverage and barriers to service use. Different qualitative and quantitative study designs that are complementary to one another provide together the most comprehensive information.

Effectiveness Evaluation: Assessing Outcome and Impact

Evaluating the effectiveness of AIDS prevention programme mes will almost always require quantitative measurements. These measurements will assess the extent to which the objectives of the programme were achieved. Effectiveness evaluation is used to answer the questions, "What outcomes were observed?" "What do the outcomes mean?," and "Does the programme make a difference?"

Taking into account the various implementation stages of HIV/AIDS prevention programme mes and the fact that, over time, new age cohorts become sexually active, it is advisable to stratify effectiveness evaluation by short-term and intermediate programme effects (programme me outcome) and long-term programme me effects (programme me impact). The examples of programme me outcome and impact measures for these different stages. Changes in HIV/AIDS-related attitudes, the reduction of risk behaviours and adoption of protective behaviours, and changes in STI rates are considered to be the most appropriate short-term or intermediate (also called proximate) outcome measures for interventions designed to reduce sexual transmission of

HIV. Long-term effects include impact on HIV/AIDS trends, sustainability issues, and improved societal response.

Outcome and impact evaluation is intimately connected with process evaluation. Process information can help the evaluator to understand how and why interventions have achieved their effects and, perhaps, what is actually making the difference. Examining outcome/impact indicators without assessing the process of programme me implementation could lead to erroneous conclusions regarding the effectiveness of the intervention.

Programme me goals and objectives have to be carefully defined to allow the selection of appropriate outcome and impact measures to assess the effectiveness of an AIDS prevention programme me . Effectiveness evaluation is generally based on indicators that provide quantitative value from which the outcome and impact of interventions can be measured. Because multiple interventions working synergistically together are most effective in producing behaviour change, surveys should not be typically designed to capture the effects of one single intervention. Rather, they should be designed to measure behavioural trends in population groups who are exposed to combined interventions. The evaluation of one intervention is usually conducted through rigorous and expensive controlled trials.

Cost-effectiveness Analysis

Cost-effectiveness analysis also measures programme me effectiveness, but expands the analysis by adding a measure of programme me cost per unit of effect (for example, per number of HIV infections averted). By comparing the costs' and consequences of various interventions, cost analyses and cost effectiveness estimates can assist in priority setting, resource allocation decisions, and programme me design. "Guidelines for Performing

Cost-effectiveness Analysis of HIV/AIDS Prevention and Care Programme me mes" provides more detail on this type of evaluation.)

The Attribution Dilemma: Are Observed Changes a Result of Prevention Interventions?

The ultimate goal of any HIV prevention programme me is to reduce the number of new infections. Programme me evaluation is intrinsically complex, however, due to the temporal evolution of epidemics and our poor understanding of how different behaviours and epidemiologic factors influence epidemic patterns as they move from an epidemic phase to an endemic state. Several factors unrelated to intervention effects can contribute to the observed stabilisation or decreases in the prevalence or incidence of HIV in a given setting. They include:

— mortality, especially in mature epidemics;
— saturation effects in populations at high risk;
— behavioural change in response to the experience of HIV/AIDS among friends and relatives;
— differential migration patterns related to the epidemic; and
— sampling bias and/or errors in data collection and analysis.

Determining whether observed changes in HIV incidence and prevalence are a reflection of the natural history of the epidemic or due to intervention effects is a critical evaluation issue. This is particularly true when evaluating behaviour changes in the face of growing numbers of people with AIDS-related illnesses because there is evidence that secular trends toward risk reduction will occur. For example, having a friend or relative with HIV/AIDS may influence adolescents to delay the onset of sexual relations or motivate those with non-regular sex partners to use condoms. Human sexual behaviour is influenced and shaped by many factors and exposure to an HIV prevention programme me is only one of them.

The question of whether behaviour changes can be attributed to prevention programme me mes, especially in countries with advanced HIV epidemics, has created some friction between stakeholders and programme me implementers at the field level. Their different perspectives on this issue also reflect fundamental differences regarding the criteria for judging the process of programme me evaluation itself. From a public health perspective, it may not matter whether the observed changes are due to a particular intervention. What is most important is that sexual practices have become safer and HIV infection should subsequently decrease.

From the cost-effectiveness or policy perspective, however, it is important to determine what caused the observed changes in sexual behaviour. If the changes would have occurred without a particular intervention that was designed to contribute to the observed changes, the costs of the intervention could be considered as resources better spent on something more useful4. Prevention programme me mes are under growing pressure to estimate which approaches work best for specific target populations in different epidemiologic settings with a given level of inputs in order to allocate resources in a cost-effective manner. Effectiveness evaluation, therefore, is critical because it can answer a basic question, "Does the programme me make a difference?"

A vexing task of assessing programme me effectiveness is to disentangle the attributable affects of a prevention programme me from the gross outcome and impact observed. Such estimates can be made with varying degrees of plausibility, but not with certainty. A general principle applies here: The more rigorous the research design, the more convincing the resulting estimate6. A hierarchy of evidence based on the study design can be established that reflects the degree of certainty in concluding that a given proportion of the observed changes in behaviour is attributable to the intervention programme me and is not the result of other factors.

A ranking of different study designs according to their decreasing strength of evidence. Non-experimental observational methods with no control groups have been routinely used in behavioural outcome evaluations. It is important to recognize, however, that a before-and-after evaluation design with no comparison groups may be useful for assessing a prevention programme me 's proficiency in delivering services, but it is not a very convincing design to measure programme me effectiveness. The inference of cause and effect from such a design is problematic because competing explanations for across-time behavioural changes cannot be ruled out.

In some situations, the evaluation could assess "exposure" to an intervention programme me or a specific element, and determine the extent of the association of that exposure with the desired outcome. This method, however, can be limited in its utility by factors such as lack of association of services or products with the intervention and inaccurate reporting by respondents of their participation in the intervention.

The interpretation of programme me evaluation data should always be approached with caution. In most situations, the programme me and evaluation process as a whole is not a rigorously controlled experimental trial. The ability of an evaluation to precisely determine the true extent of a programme me 's effectiveness is often limited by time, resources, and the lack of a rigorous design. Many factors can confuse or confound the results measured, and biases can be introduced by a range of factors inherent to the problem of HIV/AIDS, the available measurement options, and those conducting the evaluation. One of the most difficult questions to answer in any evaluation is that of attributing any measured effect to the programme me being evaluated. Defining the web of interacting and overlapping influences is extremely difficult, and is one of the reasons why so many programme me mes have difficulty attributing results to their actions. At some point, we need to stop worrying about attribution in such settings and focus on monitoring the changes as they occur.

The Role of Triangulation

Triangulation can be achieved through using multiple data sources, different researchers, multiple perspectives to interpret a single set of data, or multiple methods applied to a single programme me , problem, or issue. In the absence of rigorous controlled trials, data triangulation procedures must be applied to substantiate a link between interventions and observed behaviour changes. For example, process evaluation data on condom sales, the intensity of peer education, or the quality and coverage of media campaigns can be combined with an analysis of behavioural outcome data to provide an understanding of the process through which an intervention has achieved its effects. Results from behavioural surveys should be analysed together with findings from qualitative evaluation research that is carried out in sub-samples of surveyed target populations. Such research can include focus group discussions, key informant interviews, and rapid ethnographic studies. This type of analysis will allow a more appropriate interpretation of observed outcome data because they are the likely results of the aggregate effects of multiple interventions as well as environmental and personal factors.

Many of the areas that need to be measured to evaluate HIV/AIDS programme me mes are sensitive and very personal in nature, such as sexual behaviours or personal attitudes toward pérsons with HIV/AIDS. Validity and reliability are critical issues for sexual behaviour research because the behaviours cannot be directly observed. Self-reports of sexual behaviours in the absence of additional evidence are often considered invalid and unreliable by stakeholders for whom such data are sensitive and run against firmly held cultural norms.

One of the best methods for promoting reliability and validity, therefore, is to triangulate behavioural data with all other available and relevant biological, behavioural, and process data to explain more comprehensively the context in which risk behaviours take place. "Assessing the Validity and Reliability of Self-reported Behavioural Data," provides more detail on this issue.

Given the abundance of AIDS-related research conducted in many countries, secondary data are a source of material for triangulation. Multiple-method triangulation is probably the most common triangulation technique. Rapid ethnographic research, combining semistructured information gathering with mapping, participant observation, and in-depth interviews, is another possibility. Focus group discussions have been widely used, as have individual in-depth interviews or key informant interviews, to obtain stakeholders' (or other key individuals') opinions about target groups' behaviour. "The Role of Qualitative Data in Evaluating HIV Programme me mes," provides more information on qualitative evaluation tools.)

Finally, it is important to realise that behaviour change interventions have to be in place for sufficient amounts of time and on a large enough scale to have an impact on personal behaviour, social norms in communities, and ultimately on the epidemic. The example of Thailand shows that a focused intervention strategy implemented on a national scale can result in substantial declines in HIV incidence and prevalence in targeted populations. It is also an example of applied triangulation of data: STI/HIV trends were systematically collected by sentinel surveillance systems, and behavioural surveillance data provided the necessary supplementary information to interpret the observed epidemiological trends. There is now growing consensus that country programme me mes need to monitor risk behaviour trends together with trends in HIV infection. "Uses of Behavioural Data for Programme me Evaluation" for more on this issue.)

Choice of Indicators

One of the critical steps in designing and carrying out an evaluation of an HIV/AIDS programme me , or any programme me for that matter, is selecting appropriate indicators. This can be a fairly straightforward process if the objectives of the programme me have been clearly stated and presented in terms that define quantity, quality, and time frame of a particular aspect of the programme me . Even with well-defined objectives, however, the choice of indicators for the evaluation of many programme me mes requires careful thought and consideration of both theoretical and practical elements.

The following questions can be helpful in selecting indicators:

— Is the focus of the objective a parameter that can be measured accurately and reliably?

— Are there alternative measures that need to be considered?
— What resources (human and financial) does the indicator require?
— Are there areas for congruency, either in the content of the indicator or the means of gathering the data?
— Are there any additional measures that would help in interpreting the results of the primary objective?

Selecting indicators and setting targets is usually done during the process of programme me planning and replanning, preferably in a participatory way with the implementing agency and key stakeholders. Setting targets and benchmarks should also include information from similar types of interventions, so that the targets set are realistic from the perspective of the target population, resource allocation, and intervention type.

While the level of attainment to be measured by the indicator is not actually part of the indicator itself, it is a critical factor. The magnitude of the level to be measured affects the size of the sample of the population needed to estimate that level accurately. It may also help evaluators select additional or supplemental indicators that might assist in later interpretations of the results.

Ideally, indicators should be:

— Valid—They should measure the condition or event they are intended to measure.
— Reliable—They should produce the same results when used more than once to measure the same condition or event.
— Specific—They should measure only the condition or event they are intended to measure.

— Sensitive—They should reflect changes in the state of the condition or event under observation.

— Operational—It should be possible to measure or quantify them with developed and tested definitions and reference standards.

— Affordable—The costs of measuring the indicators also should be reasonable.

— Feasible—It should be possible to carry out the proposed data collection.

Validity is inherent in the actual content of the indicator and also depends on its potential for being measured. Reliability is inherent in the methodology used to measure the indicator and in the person using the methodology. Many familiar outcome indicators in HIV/AIDS prevention, such as measures of condom use, provide challenges to the evaluator with respect to validity and reliability.

Interpreting outcome indicators for behavioural interventions that promote safer sex is further complicated by the fact that risk behaviours are measured in relative terms. For example, percentage figures of condom use measure the proportion of sexual exposures that are considered to be safe. These may or may not reflect the absolute number of sex acts that place individuals at risk for exposure to sexual transmission. Ten percent condom use in HIV-associated sexual episodes is still "safer" than 75 percent condom use in 100 HIV-associated sex episodes (9 versus 25 unprotected HIV-associated sex acts, respectively). Therefore, in this example it also would be important to determine the frequency of condom use in absolute terms in a given risk situation. Behavioural surveys have begun to address this dilemma by collecting additional data on "always or consistent" condom use in the context of sexual episodes with non-regular partners.

The possible indicators related to different levels of programme me evaluation. The advantage of relating indicators to specific evaluation levels is that it also helps to identify opportunities for triangulating data. For example, survey data on condom use can be compared with information on condom distribution and availability in a defined intervention area. Or, available data on incident STIs, such as gonorrhea, in the surveyed population could be correlated with the condom data.

In collaboration with national and international partners, the United Nations AIDS Programme me me and the World Health Organisation (UNAIDS/WHO) have developed a standard set of indicators for country programme me mes that will refine and expand the prevention indicators (PI) developed by WHO's former Global Programme me on AIDS (GPA). Moreover, because HIV/AIDS/STI prevention and care programme me mes are affected by many factors, including political commitment, available resources, and the socio-cultural and economic context, a new approach is currently being developed to capture the overall effort of national HIV/AIDS programme me mes. The AIDS Programme me Effort Index (API) is a composite score comprised of the main components of an effective national response. The potential advantage of this instrument is that it may yield useful information on the above issues even in the absence of more rigorous monitoring and evaluation systems. Using the key informant assessment approach, it also allows an assessment of areas that are difficult to capture with more objectively measurable indicators (e.g., political support and commitment). However, major concerns have been expressed with regard to the subjectivity and reliability of the API approach. The score depends entirely on the choice of informants, and the informants are likely to change from year to year. Questions have also been raised about the utility of a single composite score in which improvements in some areas may be masked by deterioration in other areas.

Differentiating Evaluation Efforts

Because of the various constraints on time, available funds, and trained staff, programme me managers and evaluation planners must balance what is ideal or preferred against what is feasible, useful, relevant, and essential when choosing how to evaluate a particular intervention or programme me . A useful approach for differentiating evaluation efforts is to define them in three different dimensions: the individual project dimension, the country programme me dimension, and the international dimension. Using this multi-dimensional approach (individual, country, and international project) to set priorities for the degree of rigor needed to evaluate programme me mes and projects may alleviate some of the tension that arises when universal, standardized evaluation practices conflict with the objectives of individual projects.

One can think of the individual project dimension as an area of service delivery that, in most cases, does not require a rigorous research design to judge its proficiency, unless it is piloting a new intervention or responding to an unanswered research question, such as would occur with a demonstration project. Individual projects carrying out standard intervention strategies that have already been shown to be effective in other similar settings should focus their evaluation activities on formative evaluation (when needed for project planing), process evaluation, and capacity building assessment. The number of projects in relation to the different levels of evaluation efforts and reflects the current situation in programme me evaluation. The monitoring and evaluation "pipeline" illustrates that there is usually a reduced number of projects that actually warrant the evaluation of the effectiveness of their implemented prevention activities. Within the dimension of a country programme me , several categories of evaluation should be emphasized—intervention outcomes, socioeconomic impact, and changes in societal norms. The guiding principle here is that in a situation in which multiple donors are conducting multiple interventions with overlapping target groups, certain types of evaluation are not appropriate for the scope of an individual project, but rather, should be coordinated and conducted by country or regional programme me mes. Use of such an evaluation approach, especially in the area of behavioural surveys, not only saves money, but also makes sense in environments where the effects of individual projects from different donors cannot be sorted out anyway.

Country programme me evaluation includes (but is not limited to) the analysis of behavioural trends in different population groups in conjunction with an analysis of HIV/STI surveillance data; the evaluation of social marketing activities related to condoms, drugs, and services; STI case management; scoring the overall effort of the national programme me (for example, through the AIDS Programme me Effort Index); socioeconomic impact assessments; and epidemiological modeling of the country's epidemic. Countries will have different programme me mes of evaluation activities, reflecting their different information needs, which are determined by the stage of their epidemic, as well as their political and social environment, existing capacity for research, and available financial resources. Evaluation efforts on the international dimension may address still existing uncertainties about which set of prevention interventions works best, in which setting, for whom, and under what circumstances (emphasis on cost-effectiveness analysis). This type of evaluation, however, requires large-scale community-based controlled trials that are certainly beyond the scope of individual projects or even national programme me mes. Given the difficulties and high costs associated with directly measuring the impact of HIV prevention programme me mes through large-scale incidence studies, more emphasis has now been placed on developing other methods of assessing impacts, for example through modeling. "Translating Survey Data into Programme me Impact: the AVERT Model," provides more detail on one such effort. HIV/AIDS prevention and care programme me evaluation is applied socio-epidemiological research whose main purpose is to identify and solve practical problems and guide programme me managers and planners in improving the design and implementation of prevention and care activities. This perspective not only determines the role of programme me evaluation but also how an evaluation should be conducted, including the choice of indicators and levels of efforts in a given setting.

By applying different methods from several disciplines to many types of problems, programme me evaluation is a comprehensive research approach committed to meeting the needs of stakeholder groups as well as the requirements of the scientific community. This Handbook is designed to assist programme me evaluators in this critically important task. Although programme me evaluation is context specific, a comprehensive framework as outlined in this chapter is helpful in defining the questions that are to be answered by the different types of evaluation during the programme me cycle. We advocate for a utilisation-focused evaluation approach that emphasizes the interests of stakeholders as the primary intended information users. To achieve the delicate balance between practical needs and methodological desirability, it is therefore essential that programme me evaluations are planned in a participatory fashion with key stakeholders. Decisionmaking is a political process and programme me evaluators can play a major role in this process when evaluation efforts are expected to provide information of policymaking significance and relevance. Although evaluation researchers should be neutral scientific observers, there is also a need for them to assume a more active role and, if necessary, mediate between stakeholders with different and sometimes conflicting interests, perspectives, and information needs. Given the limited resources in most developing countries, assessing the effectiveness of HIV prevention programme me mes will often depart from scientifically ideal designs. In the absence of more rigorous evaluation designs, we urge programme me managers and evaluators to apply triangulation procedures using multiple complementary methods as well as different data sources. Such a triangulated analysis will provide information comprehensive enough to allow a plausible and valid interpretation of observed outcome data, such as changes in risk behaviours, because they are the likely results of the aggregate effects of multiple interventions as well as environmental and personal factors.

METHODOLOGY FOR SUMMARIZING THE EVIDENCE FOR THE PRACTICES

The Agency for Healthcare Research and Quality (AHRQ) charged the UCSF-Stanford Evidence-Based Practice Center with the task of rating or grading the patient safety practices identified and evaluated in this Compendium. The Compendium is an anthology of diverse and extensive patient safety practices, grouped by general topic (Part III, Sections A-H), and then further sorted within chapters by individual practices. Synthesis was challenging, but critical in order that readers and healthcare decision-makers could make judgments about practices to implement and/or research further. Keeping these two audiences in mind, we set 3 goals for "rating" the practices, as follows:

— Develop a framework for rating the main elements of practices within the constraints of the available literature, providing as much pragmatic information as possible to decision-makers who might endorse practices or fund further research in the area of patient safety interventions.
— Document the limitations of the rating method so that those "taking home" messages from the report understand the inherent limitations of making comparisons of a highly heterogeneous field of possible practices.
— Convey the results of the ratings in an organised, visually appealing, accessible way that ensures that our cautionary notes regarding oversimplifying the ratings are clear.

Ultimately, we aimed to weight the practices, based on the evidence, on a range of dimensions, without implying any ability to calibrate a finely gradated scale for those practices in between. Proper metrics for these comparisons (e.g., cost-effectiveness analysis) require more data than are currently available in the literature.

Data Inputs into the Practice Ratings

For each practice, information about various inputs into the final "roll-up", as we referred to our scoring of the practices, were prospectively determined. The decision about what information to attempt to gather was based on the potential expected uses of summary tables of practices. Three major categories of information were gathered to inform the rating exercise:

— *Potential Impact of the Practice*: based on prevalence

and severity of the patient safety target, and current utilisation of the practice.

— *Strength of the Evidence Supporting the Practice*: including an assessment of the relative weight of the evidence, effect size, and need for vigilance to reduce any potential negative collateral effects of practice implementation.

— *Implementation*: considering costs, logistical barriers, and policy issues.

Further clarification of the 3 categories is in order. Authors were asked to report on *prevalence and severity of the safety target* for a given practice in order to categorize the potential impact of implementing the practice. We added to this an assessment of the practice's potential impact by reviewing evidence of its *current utilisation*. If an intervention is already widely used, the room for improvement, stated in terms of additional reductions in adverse events targeted by the practice that could be achieved by wider implementation, is less than if few are currently using the practice. Thus, *potential impact of implementing the practice* is a function of the prevalence and severity of the patient safety target (e.g., medical error) and the current utilisation of the practice.

Of course the actual impact of any practice is assessable only if factors related to *evidence supporting the practice* are evaluated. Since the Compendium represents an assemblage of the evidence for patient safety practices, the instructions to authors outlined the detailed data elements related to study design and outcomes we required them to abstract from the relevant studies. This information was used to assess, in general terms, the *overall strength of the studies* for each practice. *Effectiveness* is commonly defined as the net positive effect in routine practice. Frequently the data reported in the studies related to *efficacy*, usually the net positive effect under controlled, experimental situations. The translation from efficacy to effectiveness is not straightforward if no direct evidence is available, and is therefore based on judgments about the generalizability of the specific research studies conducted. Also of key importance, and therefore abstracted from studies for use in the ratings, was the *effect size of the intervention*.

Finally, evidence-based reviews consider the *potential for harm* from a medical intervention, and authors were asked to report on any relevant evidence, as well as reasoned concerns, gleaned from the literature or from common knowledge about a practice.

To address the real-world environment and the desire by the public for action in the area of patient safety, practice chapters were designed to include information about cost and other potential barriers to *implementation*. While authors sometimes discussed cost savings or reported cost-effectiveness analyses, the focus was on the *start-up costs and annual outlays* for ongoing use of the practice. Although initial and ongoing costs are a function of local environments (e.g., size of the healthcare network or institution), possible cost savings are likely to be even more subject to local conditions (e.g., prevalence of the patient safety target). For major investment decisions, an assessment of tradeoffs is more appropriate at the local level. Our intention was simply to report "ballpark" estimates of initial and recurring costs. Separate from economic consequence of a particular practice implementation are the *political and technical considerations*.

For all of these data inputs into the practice ratings, the primary goal was to find the best available evidence from publications and other sources. Because the literature has not been previously organised with concurrent considerations of each of these areas, most estimates could be improved with further research and some are informed by only general and somewhat speculative knowledge. Where possible, in the summaries of these elements, we have attempted to highlight assessments made on the basis of limited data.

Rating Process

The 4-person Editorial Team developed a rating form that captured the patient safety target, practice description, and general rating categories (e.g., High, Medium, Low) for some of the elements described in the section above. General heuristics were specified for each category, although individual judgment for ratings was designed into the process. The form also specified comment areas to allow raters to document their specific judgments and concerns about ratings. Each chapter was independently rated by each Editor as to the practices for which there was evidence. The Editorial Team convened for 3 days to compare scores, discuss disparities, and come to consensus about ratings—both by category and summary ratings—or the reviewed practices.

Details about Decision Rules and Judgment Considerations

Potential Impact Factor

As noted above, an assessment of potential impact considered the prevalence and severity of the patient safety target, and the current utilisation of the practice being evaluated. The Editorial Team used the data from the chapters and clinical knowledge to order the potential impact as "High," "Medium," "Low," or "Insufficient Information." To qualify for the "High" score, a practice had to target a patient population of greater than 1% of hospitalized patients (about 300,000 patients per year) or target a patient safety problem that can result in death or disability. The "Low" score was used for target populations of less than 0.01% of hospitalized patients (about 3000 patient/year) who might experience reversible adverse effects if an effective practice were not available. Potential impact was deemed a "Medium" if the practice had a patient safety target that fell between the 2 other categories.

An additional decision rule was applied to the Impact rating after the initial assessment based on prevalence and severity was made. If a practice was currently widely used (>75% of hospitals), then the rating was demoted one notch (i.e., from High to Medium or Medium to Low). When this situation occurred, a notation identified that the potential impact level was impacted by its high current utilisation.

We reserved the "Insufficient Information" category for those cases where the prevalence and severity information was quite limited or where the patient safety target was ill-defined.

Evidence Supporting the Practice

Study strength, effect size on target(s), and need for vigilance due to potential harms were rated based more on judgment than pre-specified decision rules. In each case, raters documented their reasons for category choices.

For *study strength*, the level of study design and outcomes, number of studies, numbers of patients in studies, generalizability, and other methodologic issues were specified as factors to consider in weighting the relative study strength for a particular practice. Study strength could be categorized as "High," "Medium," or "Low." The actual findings of the studies were not considered when scoring study strength because this information was captured in the assessment of effect size on target. If there was minimal or no evidence about a practice, the study strength rating was "Low" and raters did not score the remaining 2 elements of the evidence supporting the practice since that might give undue "credit" to the findings. The assessment of *effect size on target(s)* was based on the relative risk reductions or odds ratios reported in the reviewed studies for evidence of effectiveness. The raters only used the findings reported in the practice chapters, and did not perform additional analyses (e.g., meta-analysis). If all studies or, in cases where there were a large number of studies, the vast majority showed a positive and appreciable effect size (i.e., greater than 15% relative risk reduction), then the positive effect size was categorized as "Robust." If there was clearly no effect or a very minimal effect (i.e., less than 5% relative risk reduction), then the positive effect size was rated as "Negligible." For findings that were considered suggestive of substantive effect, but not clearly "Robust," the category used was "Modest." The final category, "Unclear," captured those practices for which the effect size results were inconsistent. For any given practice that reduces one adverse event, it is conceivable that new problems might ensue when the practice is implemented. Thus, we subjectively rated the *concern for harm* based on the *level of vigilance* necessary to ensure that the practice, if implemented, would not result in collateral negative effects. The categories available were "Low," "Medium," and "High." Thus, a practice rated as "Low" would require little to no attentiveness to potential harms, while one rated as "High" would merit heightened monitoring for potential negative effects. These ratings were made conservatively, meaning that when in doubt, a higher vigilance category was selected.

Implementation

Assuming a 3-year lead time for implementation, patient safety practices were rated for their costs and complexity.

Costs were based on initial start-up and annual expenditures for full implementation at an average size hospital or healthcare organisation. Potential cost savings were not considered for the rating, but were reported in the practice chapters if they were documented in the literature. If a practice was expected to require expenditures of greater than about $1 million, the rating was "High." Expenditures of approximately $100,000-$1 million were categorized as "Medium." Below this level, practices were rated as "Low" in terms of cost.

The feasibility of implementation was rated by considering potential political (e.g., major shifts in who delivers care) and technical (e.g., integration of legacy and newer computer systems) obstacles. Because relatively few data exist for rating implementation complexity, we used only 2 categories, "Low" and "High," meaning relatively easy and relatively difficult. In cases in which implementation could be accomplished simply with the expenditure of dollars, we gave high cost scores but low feasibility scores.

Overall Rating for Impact/Evidence

In addition, each member of the team considered the totality of information on potential impact and evidence supporting the practice to score each on a 0 to 10 scale ("Strength of the Evidence"). For these ratings, we took the perspective of a leader of a large healthcare enterprise (e.g., a hospital or integrated delivery system) and asked the question, "If you wanted to improve patient safety at your institution over the next 3 years and resources were not a significant consideration, how would you grade this practice?" For this rating, we explicitly did *not* consider difficulty or cost of implementation in the rating. Rather, the rating simply reflected the strength of the evidence regarding the effectiveness of the practice and the probable impact of its implementation on reducing adverse events related to healthcare exposure. If the patient safety target was rated as "High" impact and there was compelling evidence (i.e., "High" relative study strength) that a particular practice could significantly reduce (e.g., "Robust" effect size) the negative consequences (e.g., hospital-acquired infections), raters were likely to score the practice close to 10. If the studies were less convincing, the effect size was less robust, or there was a need for a "Medium" or "High" degree of vigilance because of potential harms, then the rating would be lower.

Overall Rating for Research Priority

Analogously, we also rated the usefulness of conducting more research on each practice, emphasizing whether there appeared to be questions that a research programme me might have a reasonable chance of addressing successfully ("Research Priority"). Here, our "thought question" was, "If you were the leader of a large agency or foundation committed to improving patient safety, and were considering allocating funds to promote additional research, how would you grade this practice?" If there was a simple gap in the evidence that could be addressed by a research study or if the practice was multifaceted and implementation could be eased by determining the specific elements that were effective, then the research priority was high.

If the area was one of high potential impact (i.e., large number of patients at risk for morbid or mortal adverse events) and a practice had been inadequately researched, then it also would also receive a relatively high rating for research need. Practices might receive low research scores if they held little promise (e.g., relatively few patients affected by the safety problem addressed by the practice *or* a significant body of knowledge already demonstrating the practice's lack of utility). Conversely, a practice that was clearly effective, low cost and easy to implement would not require further research and would also receive low research scores.

Caveats to Ratings

For all elements assessed, divergent assessments among the 4 Editor-raters were infrequent and were discussed until consensus was reached. For each final category where differences in interpretation existed and persisted after discussion, the protocol was to document a comment about these differences. Comments were also noted when specific additional information could clarify concerns about fidelity of a specific rating. In a few cases, categories that had not been specified were created for unusual circumstances and again comments to explain the category were documented.

Rating Tables

Information Captured

Ratings were recorded on a data table, and comments were footnoted. Summarizing from the previous discussion, the various data tables appearing captured some or all of the following 11 elements and rating categories, ordered from strongest to weakest:

1. Chapter number.
2. Patient safety target(s).
3. Patient safety practice description.
4. Potential Impact: High, Medium, Low, Insufficient Information.
5. Study Strength: High, Medium, Low.
6. Effect Size: Robust, Modest, Negligible, Unclear.
7. Vigilance: Low, Medium, High.
8. Implementation cost: Low, Medium, High.
9. Implementation complexity (political, technical): Low, High.

10. Overall rating for impact/evidence: 0 to 10 (10 is highest), in 0.5 increments.
11. Overall rating for research need: 0 to 10 (10 is highest), in 0.5 increments.

Information Reported

The detailed data tables with categorisation of elements 1-9 above. Reporting specific scores for the overall ratings would imply a refinement in scoring that was neither attempted nor advisable given the nature of the information available. Where applicable, caveats to the categorisations are appended in a series of endnotes.

In rating both the strength of the evidence and the research priority, our purpose was not to report precise 1-10 scores, but *to develop general "zones" or practice groupings*. As noted earlier, better methods are available for comparative ratings *when the data inputs are available*. The relative paucity of the evidence dissuaded us from using a more precise, sophisticated, but ultimately unfeasible, approach.

The overall ratings for the "Strength of the Evidence" regarding their impact and effectiveness score, and subdivides the practices into 5 zones. Practices are listed from highest score to lowest score for each rating zone. The zones are "greatest strength" (score of 8-10), "high strength" (score of 6-7.5), "medium strength" (4-5.5), "lower impact/evidence scored practices" (score of 2-3.5), "lowest impact/evidence scored practices" (score of 0-1.5). Practices near the bottom of one zone may be just as appropriate to list near the top of the adjacent lower zone. Similarly, practices at the top of a zone may actually be more comparable to those in the adjacent higher zone. The cut-offs between zones are somewhat artificial, but allow a general and reasonable synthesis of the data on impact and evidence supporting (or negating) the effects of the practice. Readers can be confident that practices that fall in the highest zone do not belong in the lowest zone.

The overall ratings for the "Research Priority" score, and provides examples of types of research that may be helpful. Practices are categorized in 3 zones: "Further Research Likely to be *Highly* Beneficial" (scores of 7 and higher), "Further Research Likely to be Beneficial" (scores of 4 to 6.5 inclusive), and "Low Priority for Research". The chapter lists practices for each of the top two categories of research priority.

DEVELOPING AN INTEGRATED AND COMPREHENSIVE MONITORING AND EVALUATION PLAN

Incorporating evaluation at the programme me design stage is an essential element of ensuring that evaluation activities will produce useful results. Planning an intervention and designing an evaluation strategy should be inseparable activities. To ensure the relevance and sustainability of evaluation activities, project designers, in collaboration with national and local stakeholders and collaborating donors, must work in a participatory manner to develop an integrated and comprehensive evaluation plan.

The purpose of this chapter is to provide practical guidance to HIV prevention programme me managers at various levels in developing realistic integrated and comprehensive monitoring and evaluation plans. Depending on whether such plans are designed for the national or project level, they will likely consist of widely different objectives, indicators, and methodologies to obtain those indicators. National and large geographic areas, such as provinces, may focus more on impact-related measurements, such as prevalence and behavioural estimates for HIV and sexually transmitted infections (STIs). Project-level evaluation may more appropriately concentrate on process and immediate outcome indicators, such as number of people reached and STI clients treated, as well as qualitative research methods to determine whether intervention strategies are appropriate for the target audiences.

Projects at all levels, whether they consist of multiple integrated projects or single interventions, should have an evaluation plan for assessing the progress of the programme me in achieving programme me goals and objectives and informing key stakeholders and programme me designers about the results of the evaluations. Such plans will guide the design of evaluations, highlight what information or data need to be collected, and how best to collect it. Comprehensive evaluation plans should describe the overall purpose(s) of the evaluation, the specific evaluation questions to be addressed, the evaluation designs and methods to be used, what data are to be collected and how, the resources that will be necessary, who will implement the evaluation, and the basic evaluation plan timeline. They are often written to cover a 4- to 5-year period because they may involve multiple evaluative efforts on multiple interventions for multiple target populations, some of which require time to observe intervention or programme me outcomes (immediate or short-term effects), as well as overall programme me impact (long-term effects).

This chapter applies the conceptual evaluation framework offered and describes the steps involved in developing an integrated and comprehensive evaluation plan, the factors that may influence this process, and key questions that should be asked by every programme me .

Rationale for Developing an Evaluation Plan

It is often helpful in the beginning stages to review

with all stakeholders the reasons for developing a comprehensive evaluation plan. Some of the benefits that can be derived from the evaluation planning process are:

- Evaluation planning will provide programme me managers and stakeholders alike with the opportunity to assess the evaluation needs, resources, capabilities, and priorities in their area.
- Having an evaluation plan will show stakeholders how the programme me plans to be accountable for the resources they have received.
- In the process of developing the evaluation plan, existing data sources and past or concurrent evaluation activities are often identified. Capitalizing on such existing data sources and past evaluative efforts can lead to a more efficient, less redundant plan for new evaluation monies.
- Having a long-term evaluation plan can clarify future decision-making regarding evaluation priorities.
- Finally, having a comprehensive evaluation plan in place may also fav urably influence donor decision-making.

Key Elements of an Evaluation Plan

In developing an evaluation plan, a planning group should focus on the following key elements:

- Scope of the evaluation—Specifying the goals and objectives of the programme me and developing a conceptual framework (or logic model) that integrates and correlates the inputs, activities, outputs, outcomes, and impact, and establishing realistic expectations for what the evaluation will provide or show
- Methodological approach—Developing an evaluation

design, including specifying the outcome indicators or measures and the data source and plans for data analysis

— Implementation plan—Delineating activities, roles, and responsibilities, and a timetable for identified activities with realistic expectations of when data will be analysed and results will be available

— Dissemination plan for the results—Determining who will translate the results into language that is useful to programme me designers, managers, and decision makers, how findings will be disseminated (for example, written papers, oral presentations, programme me materials), and implications for setting priorities for future evaluation activities

Developing an Integrated and Comprehensive Evaluation Plan

In some cases, these elements are already in place and the task of the evaluation planning group is to pull them together into an integrated logical whole. If these elements have not been previously developed, then the following steps may be helpful in beginning an evaluation plan.

Evaluation planning generally involves several common steps. These steps are described here in a general way so as to allow for differences among programme me types, target populations, stakeholders' needs for information, and the various levels such as a national programme me , a district or provincial response, and individual projects reaching specific target groups. Throughout the process, it is important to involve the various stakeholders: programme me planners, evaluators, Ministry of Health and National AIDS Control Programme me staff, as well as donors. Involving members of the target community also helps inform the evaluation planning process. This stakeholder involvement in the early phases helps to ensure that the evaluation results will be used in the end. As Box 2-1 shows, both internal and external perspectives are critical.

Step 1: Identify Programme me Goals and Objectives

The first step involves identifying the programme me goals and objectives and establishing a programme me logic model. This is done through writing a clear statement that identifies the programme me 's goals and objectives (and sometimes sub-objectives) and describes how the programme me sees itself operating to achieve these objectives. When this is done, a programme me logic model can be easily diagrammed and used to establish an evaluation plan.

Each component of the programme me should have objectives and sub-objectives specified, and each objective and sub-objective should designate measures of success indicators that should be collected to determine progress. The programme me logic model showing sample goals, objectives, activities, indicators, and methods to obtain indicators, at both the country and project levels.

This model illustrates the way that the role of national governments in monitoring and planning HIV prevention is distinct from, yet complements, the implementing strengths of individual projects at the local level. For example, individual projects do not typically conduct impact evaluation because their impacts are typically seen in tandem with those of other projects that work synergistically at multiple levels toward the same goals. Impact evaluation is most appropriately measured in large geographic areas, such as a province or country, and examines whether the collective efforts of numerous projects are reaching their desired impacts. These impacts can be measured through the serosurveillance systems, which monitor trends in HIV and STI prevalence as well as through repeated behavioural risk surveys. Local organisations, which have direct contact with target groups through outreach, STI treatment, and care, for example, should focus their evaluation efforts on assuring quality programme me implementation as opposed to outcome or impact evaluation. This means more of a concentration on quality inputs, such as training and pretesting of communication messages, but also includes the coverage and density of interventions. This model also illustrates the length of time needed to show progress at various levels—ranging from several months for process-level accomplishments, such as staff trained, to several years fcr outcome- and impact-level goals.

If the information or data necessary to complete Step 1 are not readily available, then plans should be developed to collect them. This step concludes with a written specification of the programme me logic model, using the framework, and a general statement about priority evaluation questions to be addressed in the evaluation plan.

This last aspect—framing the evaluation questions and then setting priorities among them—is sometimes quite difficult when there are multiple stakeholders involved and resources, time, and evaluation expertise are limited. Thus, the evaluation questions may need revision later in the evaluation plan development process.

Step 2: Examine Existing Data and Past Evaluation Studies

The second step consists of identifying existing data sources as well as other evaluative activities that may have been done in the past, are ongoing, and/or may have been sponsored by other donors. At this step, evaluation planning teams should assess whether other groups are planning similar evaluations and invite them to collaborate in the planning and coordination.

Step 3: Identify Internal and External Evaluation Resources and Capacity

Identifying evaluation resources means not only identifying the funds for the evaluation, but also other types of resources, such as personnel experienced in evaluation to assist in planning and conducting the evaluation activities. It also means determining the programme me 's capacity to manage and link various databases and computer systems.

Step 4: Determine Evaluation Questions, Their Feasibility, and Appropriate Designs and Indicators

In the fourth step, evaluation experts and programme me managers clarify the priority evaluation questions, appropriate evaluation designs, outcome measures or indicators, data needs, and the methods by which this information will be collected and analysed. Practical ways for obtaining data and maintaining a data system that is sustainable and easily accessed should be discussed. An operational plan for the comprehensive evaluation plan should be developed at this step as well. Thus, this step should conclude with a revised written plan briefly outlining the evaluation questions and evaluation design, data collection methods and analysis plan, and overall timeline for the comprehensive plan.

Step 5: Plan for Disseminating and Using Evaluation Findings

The fifth step is not always performed, but should be because it is extremely useful in ensuring that evaluation findings are used to inform programme me improvement and decision-making. This step involves planning how evaluation results will be used, translated into programme me policy language, and disseminated to all relevant stakeholders and decision makers. It should also involve a feedback loop to the planners of the next evaluation and a feedback mechanism should be built in so that past lessons learned can effectively inform new efforts.

It is important that evaluation findings be translated into language that is useful for programme me designers in their efforts to improve programme me mes and that they contain implications and actions needed, if appropriate, at national and/or local levels. This fifth step is often best conducted in collaboration with individuals or groups familiar with the intervention. Evaluation results, like all messages, must be marketed and "packaged" for their target audiences. "Effective Dissemination of Data Collection Results," provides useful guidance on ways in which programme me mes can better carry out this step of the evaluation planning process.

This step is often overlooked in the planning and implementation phase of the evaluation, and often only becomes an issue when there is a problem at the end of the evaluation and someone asks the question, "How has this evaluation plan been implemented and how have the results been used to improve HIV prevention programme me mes and policy?" If there has been no plan for disseminating results and using the findings, this question often cannot be answered because the people involved in the evaluation have forgotten the details or have moved on. The lack of such a plan can undermine the usefulness of the evaluation and future activities. Inadequate dissemination also commonly leads to redundancy in evaluation efforts because others are not aware of the findings of previous evaluation efforts. It also reinforces a negative stereotype about evaluations, which is that they are not really intended to help improve programme me mes. For all these reasons, programme me mes should include a plan for disseminating evaluation findings in their overall evaluation plan.

Using Technical Support

After an evaluation plan has been developed following the above steps and including the essential elements described, programme me managers are faced with the question, "How are we really going to implement this plan?" Clearly, the success of the plan depends on the technical capacity of the programme me and its associated staff to carry out the evaluation activities. This invariably requires evaluation technical assistance. Evaluation expertise typically can be provided by individuals internal or external to the Ministry of Health or National AIDS Control Programme me . Such individuals usually have knowledge and training in the theories and methods of applied programme me evaluation. Potential evaluation experts might be found in planning and evaluation units in the Ministry of Health, local academic institutions, non-governmental organisations, and private consulting firms.

Technical capacity at the field level to design, implement, and maintain data collection systems is important to ensure the uninterrupted flow of consistent data. Participation of local people with a vested interest in the results should occur throughout the process of planning, data collection, analysis, and feedback.

Some traditional methodologies in evaluation, such as surveys on knowledge, attitudes, behaviours, and practices, may not always be appropriate for all evaluations. Technical guidance is especially important in complex evaluation designs, such as quantitative surveys where sampling designs, sample sizes, and questionnaire design must be carefully determined.

Implementing the Plan, Checking Progress, and Deciding When to Make Mid-Course Corrections

A comprehensive evaluation plan as described above

has multiple components, some of which need to occur in a sequential fashion. Additionally, sufficient evaluation resources (both human and fiscal) for the entire plan are often not available at the launching of the plan. Thus, implementing components of the evaluation plan in phases is not only logical and practical, it is also essential.

Carrying out and completing components of the evaluation in phases provides the opportunity for the evaluation planning group to assess how well the evaluation plan is working. Sometime after the group completes the first or second evaluation activity, the plan may need some revisions or corrections. It is helpful for the group to spend time at this point ensuring that the plan is still useful. This process need not be very involved. The group can begin by discussing the following questions:

— Are the evaluation activities going as planned?

— Are the evaluation questions that were initially posed being sufficiently answered? Are other data needed to answer these questions? How can such data be obtained?

— Do the evaluation questions themselves need reframing? Have other evaluation questions arisen since the initial planning that need to be incorporated into the plan at this point?

— Are there any methodological issues that need addressing or changes that need to be made to the evaluation designs? Are there any other factors, practical or political, that need to be considered in the evaluation activities yet to be implemented?

— Are any changes in the plan needed at this time? How will these changes be made? Who will implement them?

— Is the right mix of personnel and fiscal resources still available to carry out the rest of the evaluation plan?

— How are findings from the evaluation activities so far being used and disseminated? Does anything need to be done to enhance their application to programme me mes?

This assessment is most helpful if it occurs annually throughout the plan. If the plan is kept current and relevant, it will help ensure the usefulness and quality of the remaining components. It will also foster the overall success and usefulness of all of the evaluation activities by the end of the project period. Reviewing the evaluation plan and doing mid-course corrections as needed also facilitates the connection between the evaluation activities and the programme me mes as well as the design of subsequent plans.

Although projects may differ greatly in their scope, target audience, objectives, and activities, they all need to include realistic and comprehensive monitoring and evaluation plans. Incorporating evaluation in the programme me planning and design phase is essential to ensuring that evaluation activities will produce useful results. Involving national and local stakeholders and collaborating donors is an essential element of successful evaluation activities, as is broad dissemination of results.

This chapter has described a five-step process to guide programme me managers in developing evaluation plans that describe the purpose of the evaluation, the specific questions to be addressed, the evaluation designs and methods, the resources that will be needed, the people involved, and the timeline. It also has presented a programme me logic model that evaluation planners can use as a framework for laying out the evaluation plan. By following these steps, programme me planners can greatly enhance their chances of conducting evaluations that are useful, informative, and timely for HIV prevention efforts.

PRACTICES RATED BY STRENGTH OF EVIDENCE

After rating practices on a metric for potential impact, and on the strength of the evidence, we grouped them into 5 categories (Tables 57.1-57.5). These categorisations reflect the current state of the evidence. If a practice that addresses a highly prevalent or severe patient safety target receives a low rating on the impact/evidence scale, it may be because the strength of the evidence base is still weak due to lack of evaluations. As a result the practice is likely to show up at a high level on the research priority scale. However, if the practice has been studied rigorously, and there is clear evidence that its effectiveness is negligible, it is rated at the low ends of both the "strength of the evidence" (on impact/effectiveness) scale and the "research priority" scale.

A designation for the cost and complexity of implementation of the practice is included. The ratings for implementation are "Low," which corresponds to low cost and low complexity (e.g., political, technical); "Medium," which signifies low to medium cost and high complexity, *or* medium to high cost and low complexity; and "High," which reflects medium to high cost and high complexity.

Several practices are not included in the tables because they were not rated. This set of practices have long histories of use outside of medicine, but have not yet received enough evaluations for their potential healthcare applications:

— Promoting a Culture of Safety.

- — Use of Human Factors Principles in Evaluation of Medical Devices.
- — Refining Performance of Medical Device Alarms (e.g., balancing sensitivity and specificity of alarms, ergonomic design).
- — Fixed Shifts or Forward Shift Rotations.
- — Napping Strategies.

3

Critical Access Hospitals: Administrative Aspects

ADMINISTRATION IN CRITICAL ACCESS HOSPITALS

Strong hospital administration is vital to the success of critical access hospitals (CAHs). Tracking Team members from the six collaborating centers visited 40 hospitals over the first two years of this project, and found a generally competent cohort of administrators and administrative teams who had led their organisations through CAH conversion.

The Rural Hospital Flexibility Programme (Flex Programme) requires local implementation within each participating rural community. The purpose of this chapter is to discuss the importance of hospital administration to the success of local implementation efforts, and to explore policy options to support the effectiveness of local leadership.

Tracking Team members believe there is an important relationship between successful hospitals and strong, knowledgeable administrators who create partnerships with the communities in which their hospitals are located. We were not surprised that the first round of CAH conversions was accomplished by administrators who learned of the programme earlier than many of their peers, because of strong connections with their hospital associations and/or by reading national publications. Many of these individuals were willing to take some risks, and could technically navigate the largely uncharted waters of conversion protocols.

Literature Review

There is not an extensive literature describing the roles and practices of successful rural hospital administrators. In 1996, Stephen Mick discussed the relationship between strategic management activity and the financial performance of rural hospitals. He noted the "rough consensus" that emerged over the previous decade that rural hospitals are not particularly able or adept market players (although there are exceptions). He concluded that if states or the nation want to nurture a network of thriving acute care hospitals, policy makers should not rely on an approach that is based entirely on the "individual strategic actions of each rural hospital." He advocated a "coherent federal and state policy, with appropriate levels of underwriting and subsidies, that acknowledges that rural hospitals require special considerations and subsidies." Presumably programmes such as the Rural Hospital Flexibility Programme would constitute such considerations and subsidies. Mick concluded, "Despite the findings of our own research and that of others, the fact is that most rural hospitals have *not* closed and have managed to keep going despite mediocre financial performance." He writes, "Rural administrators manage quite well considering their resource poor environments," and points out that they are particularly adept at finding funding sources from their communities to keep facilities open.

Despite Mick's recommendation that rural health policy avoid reliance on the individual hospital administrator's strategic initiative, most national and state policies have done just that. Individual hospital administrators and their governing boards have been responsible for the success or failure of America's rural hospitals. In contrast, it is the rare urban or suburban hospital that sinks or swims depending on the performance of a single administrator.

In Washington State, a long-time and well-respected rural hospital administrator, Gordon McLean, has likened the rural hospital to the bumblebee. "There is no logical or aerodynamic reason why a creature so designed should be able to fly." The implication is that it is the sheer death-defying will power and magical talent of administrators, boards, clinical staff and communities that keeps these animals aloft.

Hanh Trinh wrote another article on strategic management of rural hospitals in 1999 in which he concluded, "some rural hospitals...like organisations in general, are able to pursue and alter a variety of strategies under harsh environmental/organisational constraints." In particular, the types of changes required by CAH conversion include formulating integration strategies, which Trinh found to require complicated coordination among organisations. While he did not examine the role of hospital administrators in particular in carrying through these strategies, these individuals are clearly critically important to the process.

Rita Harmata examined the link between planning and performance in her 1997 article in the *Journal of Rural Health*. She noted that "community-wide planning activities were important...in developing the will and ability to act" and that "The planning process should be broadly inclusive to generate the political support for implementing the plan." Clearly, it is up to hospital administrators and their boards to organise and invest in such planning activities.

In support of Harmata's findings, Hagopian et al (1997) reported that "strong" rural hospitals were more likely to have one or more board retreats per year, conduct an annual review of mission and goals, use active board committees, apply recruitment plans for new board members, and budget for continuing board education. These investments in governance require strong administration. Mick and colleagues (1994) thoroughly examined various rural hospital strategic initiatives to discover what correlated with financial performance, and found no consistent connections. This finding forced him to conclude: "Explanations may reside in a broader formulation of strategy. Other indicators probably need to be examined, and they include measures of community support, private fund raising, increased local tax support, political finesse, and the like...." These factors are all related to the skill and talent of local hospital administrators.

Keith Mueller and colleagues reported in 1999 that rural hospital reactions to marketplace changes varied from defensive (deflecting the "evils of managed care") to welcoming (managed care viewed as opportunities to improve). A key factor in explaining the differences is "local leadership," which includes the hospital administrator.

A review of rural hospital CEO careers in 1994 showed that 74 percent of Washington State administrators had advanced degrees (compared to 93% for urban hospitals). Twenty percent of the state's hospital administrators had administered only rural hospitals, and 17 percent had begun in urban hospitals, but moved to rural ones. Only six percent moved from rural to urban hospitals.

Survey Findings

We hypothesized that CAH administrators would be more likely than their non-converting peers to be:

— "Early adopter" types, more involved in their associations and more political,
— Part of bigger systems that promote conversion, or
— Financially desperate.

We believe our site visits support the first hypothesis. Many of the hospital administrators we met were on their state hospital association boards or involved in national association activities, and had learned about the CAH programme opportunity well before their peers. We do not have evidence to support our second hypothesis. The survey of hospital administrators conducted by the University of Minnesota for the Tracking Team in the winter of 2000 did not indicate that early converters were any more likely to be members of hospital systems than later converters. Our third hypothesis was found to be likely true, although the evidence is far from conclusive. Hospitals that converted prior to the year 2000 were more likely to report financial losses (81% of them) than those who converted during the year 2000 (73% of them), according to the administrator survey. This supports our hypothesis that early converters might have been more financially desperate than later converters. State office of rural health staff are also telling us that later converters in some states are larger, more stable rural hospitals.

Administrator Turnover

Tracking Team members were aware that administrator turnover can be a serious barrier to strategic decision making, stability and progress in general. Some small hospitals can have significant turnover. This coupled with the fact that the boards that recruit and employ them are highly variable in their ability to steer these organisations, hospital survival is dependent largely on the quality of a few leaders. There were three notable findings from the administrator survey with relation to administrator turnover:

— *Hospitals in a more desperate financial condition were more likely to have had more than two administrators during the last five years.*

Among the 50 hospitals with high turnover in the last five years, 90 percent were in desperate financial straits. Among the 114 with lower turnover, 70 percent were financially "desperate." Among the desperate, 36 percent had high turnover, compared to 13 percent among the "not desperate." (p=.006, n=164)

— *Hospitals with lower turnover tended to be in communities that were rated "supportive" by the administrators.*

While 62 percent of the low-turnover hospitals were in reportedly "high support" communities, only 46 percent of high-turnover hospitals were in "high support" communities. Among "high support" communities, 75 percent had low turnover, compared to 58 percent low turnover in low support communities. (p=.079, n=215)

— *Communities that support their hospitals with tax dollars have lower turnover in their hospital administration.*

While 37 percent of communities providing no tax support had high turnover, only 25 percent of those with tax support experienced high turnover. Fifty-six percent of high-turnover hospitals received no tax support, and 57 percent of low-turnover hospitals received tax support. (p=.076, n=215)

Board Relationships

CAH administrators in general tended to be more likely to praise their boards than bemoan their lack of competence. In an open-ended question, we asked administrators to name the major strengths and weaknesses of the hospital organisation in governance, administration and infrastructure. While 37 administrators named a weakness in relation to their boards, there were 86 administrators who said their boards were sources of real strength for the hospital.

Hospital Strengths and Weaknesses

Hospital administrators reported that their major problems were:

— Inpatient census
— Medicaid
— *Recruiting physicians*
— Medicare
— Modernizing
— Cash flow
— State legislatures

They responded that their main strengths were:

— Board and administration
— Quality of care
— Ancillary services
— Relations with the state hospital association
— Relations with the state office of rural health
— Network relationships

A review of these lists reveals that:

— No financial strengths were listed
— Only 27 percent listed reputation as a strength
— Only 36 percent reported scope of services was a strength
— Few have initiatives planned related to reputation or scope of services

Strategic Planning

Two-thirds of CAH chief executive officers (CEOs) have strategic plans for their facilities. While this is the good news, the bad news is that a third do not even have such plans. Of the plans in place, the focus is on:

— Modernizing equipment and physical plant; 50 percent
— Recruiting staff; 50 percent
— Recruiting physicians; 45 percent
— Improving collections; 41 percent
— Expanding scope of services; 36 percent
— Improving reputation; 27 percent

Administrator Characteristics

While we can profile administrators with regard to various characteristics such as education, we found no data to suggest that any of these characteristics are associated with hospital strengths or weaknesses.

Results from the survey regarding CEOs are as follows:

— Just over a third of the administrators (35%) were promoted from within the facility to the CEO job.
— The average administrator had held his or her job almost six years.
— The average hospital had two administrators during the past five years.
— Almost a third of hospitals (30%) had more than two administrators during the last five years.
— Half the administrators ended their formal educations with an undergraduate college degree.
— Sixteen percent of the CEOs had an MHA, thirteen percent had an MBA, and two percent held MPH degrees.

— The average age of administrators was 48, and 65 percent were male.
— Forty-one percent of the CEOs reported their relationships with physicians to be excellent, and forty-three percent indicated that their relationships were very good (84% excellent or good).

Site Visit Findings

We visited at least three communities where new administrators during the last one to five years appear to have played a significant role in rescuing their hospitals from closure. In one community, there was a 20-year history of administrative turnover-ten administrators in twenty years. As might be predicted, this turnover was coupled with a reputation for poor quality care. The reputation seemed to be related to the group of physicians associated with the hospital. One physician, in particular, admitted many patients to the hospital but was known to have poor behaviour with staff and patients and was not well respected. His financial value to the hospital, however, made the board and administrators reluctant to confront the problem. The physical plant had not been updated, and staff salaries lagged.

This city-owned facility was being run by a management company that provided both the CEO and the chief financial officer (CFO). There was a glitch, though. The management company was owned by the CEO assigned to this hospital, and the financial turnaround he was engineering seemed to be generated by unsustainable increases in the price structure. An audit revealed questionable practices, and the CFO, who had instigated the audit, was retained as administrator after dismissal of the management company. The new CEO convinced the board to suspend the privileges of the difficult physician whose admitting practices were suspect.

The turnaround for the facility came after this difficult period. The board made courageous decisions to restructure the hospital's leadership and make way for new physician staff. The new administrator hired seven new physicians over the past two years, and brought lab, ultrasound, physical therapy, and other diagnostic technologies back to the facility after they had been contracted out by previous administrators. The new administrator also convinced the board to convert to CAH status as part of the general package of reforms brought about by the turnaround. The $600,000 debt related to the previous administrator's price structure was repaid to Medicare, and the hospital has been breaking even ever since. Though the hospital's success can be attributed to new and effective leadership, the CAH programme provided a tool for that leadership to use in the effort to keep the hospital viable.

Another hospital we visited is publicly-owned and had a history of administrative turnover, closed briefly in 1989, and was in danger of closing again five or six years ago. Prior to the arrival of the current administrator, the emergency room (ER) had been closed for several months. The current CEO, who arrived in the fall of 1999, is the seventeenth or eighteenth employed by the hospital in the past 25 years. Historically, the board engaged in micro-management (wherein the board manages at too detailed a level, which disempowers their CEOs and contributes to their not being able to focus on important strategic issues), a behaviour of boards known to contribute to turnover or other dysfunction. One previous administrator had no experience in health care, but was a local elected official. She was hired during a time of serious financial distress for the facility. This individual, described as "dictatorial and confrontational," was alleged to have used retirement fund contributions during periods of cash flow difficulty. Lawsuits were filed by staff members. A variety of consultants were hired during this CEO's tenure, despite the poor reputations of these consultants in the industry.

Upon the termination of this administrator, the board managed to recruit an experienced and competent CEO who came recommended by nearby hospitals. His first priorities upon arrival were to improve employee morale and recruit physicians. The hospital started by recruiting a family physician and a nurse practitioner and now has a physician medical director who covers the ER, five additional new physicians, and a nurse practitioner.

The new administrator made himself visible in the community, and continues to make an effort to speak to community groups such as Rotary and Kiwanis. This was considered important to attracting patients back to the hospital after a long period of turmoil. Another effort of the administrator is to network with other hospitals and four American Indian tribes in the region. The hospital is also working closely with the local health department. Our site visitors felt that one of the reasons this administrator has been so successful was because of the strong collaboration among the four competent hospital administrators in the region, who have elected to be mutually supportive. These hospitals form a mini-network within a larger hospital network, and have found many creative ways to collaborate. For example, a project with the nearby American Indian tribe is using casino profits to purchase equipment and place the equipment at the most logical hospital.

In a third example, we visited a hospital that had been sold to a religiously-affiliated chain a couple of decades ago. The chain went through some difficulties with poor administration itself, and the hospital was threatened with closure. In the mid-1990s, local government entities created a consortium to purchase back the facility at a price of $2 million, but not before it lost its Joint Commission on the Accreditation of Healthcare Organisations (JCAHO) accreditation and was put on probation by HCFA. Also during this time, three physicians lost their licenses (e.g., for substance abuse and fraud). Relations with the Federally Qualified Health Centers (FQHCs) in town deteriorated during this time, as the physicians were on staff there as well.

The current administrator was hired in the midst of this turmoil. She is one of the longest-term administrators in the state at this point, and is running one of the most isolated hospitals in a stand-alone arrangement. She found one loyal and competent physician to stand by the hospital, and recruited several additional J-1 waiver physicians and opened a Rural Health Clinic. The hospital is now planning a building replacement project, and is feeling quite optimistic. This was another example of an administrator who was active in her association and kept abreast of national affairs as they relate to rural hospitals. This meant she was ready when the CAH programme came along, and seized the opportunity for her facility.

The state offices of rural health we visited had mixed reports on the state of hospital administration in their states. One state office reported a fair amount of rotation among administrators at CAHs and other small rural hospitals. About half of the individuals were reported to be "adequate " and the rest were "well over their heads." Confirming our hypothesis about the importance of effective administration in the decision to convert to CAH, the state office representatives reported that most of the struggling administrators were at facilities that have not converted and do not have plans to do so.

Tracking Team members were unlikely to visit hospital administrators who were in serious trouble. We usually selected sites on the recommendation of state office of rural health staff, who understood the goals of our project and were unlikely to recommend visiting hospitals that were failing•or had poor administration. One site we visited in Year 01, however, was selected because it was one of only two available CAHs to visit in the state at that time. When we called this hospital to check back during Year 02, we discovered the first administrator had died while on the job several months after our visit. The new administrator seemed like a competent individual, squeezed out of his previous hospital administration job when the hospital was sold to a for-profit organisation. He has not moved to the community where his new job is, however, and commutes from across the state a few days a week. His new position is very challenging, since the hospital has nearby competition (there is another small hospital in the county), suppliers were requiring cash to deliver goods because of a history of bankruptcy, and one of the two local physicians had just left. The nursing home on the hospital campus shares no services with the hospital and is privately owned by a local physician. The health department competes with the hospital by operating a Rural Health Clinic. Relations with the network hospital have not progressed, and the emergency medical system (EMS) operates at a basic-only level.

While this situation would seem disastrous to most, our intrepid interim administrator saw it as an interesting challenge. He made himself a list of short-term strategies, which included converting the ER to an on-call basis to save the huge fees being charged by the staffing agency, recruiting a new physician, applying for Health Professional Shortage Area (HPSA) status, applying for financing to upgrade radiology, and establish occasional specialty clinics.

These changes coupled with the increased CAH reimbursement are moving this hospital closer to financial stability and improving quality of care.

The lesson from this situation is to underscore Stephen Mick's finding, cited earlier: despite the odds, the vast majority of these hospitals remain open, driven by compelling missions and administrators with guts and gumption. With a little support and direction from a state office of rural health or hospital association, these administrative jobs might be a little more manageable and might retain people in a ratio better than the current average of two administrators in five years.

Policy Implications

The Center for Health Care Leadership collaborated with Arthur Andersen Consulting, and Dr. Stephen Shortell of the University of California at Berkeley, to publish findings of a study on hospital quality that included a significant component on hospital leadership. The findings were that the following are factors that relate to improving quality and value (and they all depend on administrative leadership):

- — How does the administrator relate to the board? (Does s/he share information, decision making?)
- — Is there a customer-service ethic? (a culture of service, quality and value?)
- — Are physicians an active, positive part of the team? Does the administrator relate well to physicians?
- — Are performance incentives aligned with goals?
- — Does the culture seem open? Is there a spirit of teamwork and information sharing?

As we learned in the literature review on rural hospital administration, however, much of the work on hospital leadership is oriented towards managers of large urban or suburban facilities. The guidelines above would certainly relate to rural facilities as well as urban ones, but there are few organisations that work on upgrading the quality of rural hospital administration. This is not a serious focus of either university training programmes, health system associations or government, although there have been a few isolated efforts.

One of the benefits of the Flex Programme is that it allows grantees at the state level to bring together hospital administrators for CAH meetings, where discussion and education can take place about current trends in the profession, common problems, and the celebration of successes. It has also allowed state office representatives and consultants to work directly on site in communities with hospital boards, facilitate networking among providers within towns, and promote networking among hospital administrators within a region.

Some of the activities that state offices of rural health and the Federal Office of Rural Health Policy (FORHP) may want to explore as they create opportunities for administrators to gain continuing education include:

- Team building and communication
- Strategic planning
- Assessing community needs
- Improving governance
- Strengthening finances
- Networking with other health providers in the same community
- Networking with health providers in other communities
- Improving quality of care
- Working with physicians

A focus group we conducted with a group of CAH administrators in Washington State (June 2001) indicated that they very much appreciated having a new peer group with which to interact, and were eager for learning opportunities offered by the state office of rural health that they could attend together. As discussed above in the results sections, the hospital association involvement, financial stability, community support, application of inventive programmes, and the like are all associated with CAH success. We believe that many of these CEO relationships and skills are being enhanced through Flex Programme activities.

CRITICAL ACCESS HOSPITALS AND COMMUNITY DEVELOPMENT

While the Federal Office of Rural Health Policy has not made "community development" one of its five specific goals for the Rural Hospital Flexibility Programme (Flex Programme), it has certainly encouraged states to support such activity in rural communities and has funded efforts at local, state and national levels to promote it.

"Community development" is a term with multiple meanings, depending on the context and the motivation. These activities can include everything from "health fairs" to "needs assessments" to "community-based strategic planning." We would argue that initiatives that actively engage community members ("stakeholders") in *decision making* related to health care can be characterized as meaningful community development.

These decision-making activities usually bring together members of a community to engage in strengthening and expanding their health care systems. Typically, citizens are engaged in assessing the strengths and weaknesses of their health care system, and then work with each other to make improvements. Implementation of plans generally involves all parts of the health system, from public health and mental health to traditional and alternative providers to social support organizations.

The most obvious motivation for hospitals to engage in community development activities is that it builds market share. By involving community members in identifying community needs, planning, fundraising, improving reputation, marketing, recruiting workforce, and expanding services, hospitals gain visibility and credibility, typically resulting in increased utilization. Building support from community leaders also provides opportunities for hospitals to gain support for tax subsidies through ongoing levies or capital bonds as well as increased private fund raising capacity through gifts, endowments, and capital campaigns. In addition, all of these types of activities help to ensure that the hospital is in touch with its community and meeting its needs.

As hospitals consider critical access hospital (CAH) status, many view conversion as an opportunity to engage the community's health care providers and consumers in a discussion about the local health care system as a whole.

Background

The National Rural Health Association (NRHA) published a report in 1995 summarizing a variety of approaches and techniques for community rural health development that were developed around the country by universities, state offices of rural health, Area Health Education Centers (AHECs), private consultants and other rural health advocates over the previous decade. That publication notes:

Reimbursement policies, provider shortages, and economic and population trends were blamed for the health system failures of the last decade, but new research shows that the level of community awareness of, confidence in and support for the local health care delivery mechanisms play critical roles in sustaining community services.

Many of the community development activities featured in that report were launched at a time when rural hospitals were particularly threatened by having to adapt to prospective payment systems in the mid-1980s. The publication classified the various activities into three models: comprehensive, planning and self-help. The comprehensive model approach includes "Community Health Services Development," developed at the University of Washington through a grant from the W.K. Kellogg Foundation, and subsequent grants from the Northwest Area Foundation. The Community Decision Making model was developed at the Mountain States Group in Boise, Idaho, under sponsorship from the Area Health Education Center. The Rural Health Transition Model, funded by the Blandin Foundation, was developed by Minnesota's Center for Rural Health.

The planning models (second approach) were mostly single-state based, and included Hometown Health, developed in Iowa as a joint effort of the Center for Rural Health at the Iowa Department of Public Health, and programmes at Iowa State University. Alabama County Health Councils were the brainchild of the University of Alabama and Auburn University. Community Wellness Councils were local planning organizations created by county extension agents and supported by the University of Georgia. The Missouri Rural Innovative Institute was another Kellogg-funded effort that also worked through extension, AHECs, and the University of Missouri. Not mentioned in the NRHA publication is the PATCH (Planned Approach to Community

Health) programme, described as a process that involves and enables members of a community to organize and mobilize members, collect and use local area data, set health priorities, select and implement appropriate interventions, and perform process and impact evaluation. PATCH was popularized in Nebraska and Wyoming, among other places.

The third approach is self-help. Community Voices was another Kellogg Foundation effort at North Carolina A&T State University that focused primarily on disadvantaged rural communities in the south. "Working Together for Rural Action," another Northwest Area Foundation effort, was developed by the University of North Dakota Center for Rural Health. Community Oriented Primary Care is another effort in this category, with a particular initiative funded by NRHA and Kellogg to demonstrate the value of combining epidemiology and primary health care skills to systematically identify and address the major health care needs, problems and concerns of rural communities.

Following these efforts, which spanned from the mid-1980s to the mid-1990s and beyond, the Federal Office of Rural Health Policy (FORHP) committed to a national community development effort in some of America's most economically-deprived rural communities. "Community Solutions for Rural Health" was implemented in three waves, starting first with communities in the Southeast states. Leaders from the community development efforts of the previous decade were recruited to design a programme and train local "encouragers," who implemented local projects. This effort was evaluated and described in another NRHA publication.[4]

The next (and current) wave of related activities, "Operation Rural Health Works," was developed at Oklahoma State University.[i] In this project, a methodology has been developed to assess the economic impact of the health system on rural communities (economic multiplier values are calculated). This FORHP-funded effort is training state offices of rural health and other interested parties to adopt the approach, develop the information, and bring it to communities where local decision making can be performed.

Community development is not easily described, nor does it have a large or powerful national constituency or following. There are national interests, however, that can be achieved most effectively and efficiently through community development initiatives. One of these is quality of care. The recent Institute of Medicine's report on quality[5] has encouraged a more coordinated health care system nationally. Rural communities are well positioned to implement and demonstrate strategies quickly and effectively as their systems are small and can be agile.

State Offices of Rural Health

When we investigated community development activities spawned by the Flex Programme, we encountered the inevitable problem of defining what qualifies as serious community development activity. Some of the state offices and hospitals would characterize very limited efforts as "community development," while others would only include activities similar to those characterized in the 1995 NRHA report, summarized above.

Thirty state offices of rural health ("state offices") responded to a Flex Programme Tracking Team e-mail survey regarding how communities are engaging in health system development coincident with CAH conversion. Eighty-three percent of these state office respondents indicated they were using some of their Flex Programme grant dollars to conduct, facilitate or promote community development activities in CAH locales. Two-thirds of these state offices reported that "many" communities were taking advantage of conversion as an opportunity to engage in development, and 86 percent of the states were convinced that these activities were valuable.

Fewer than half the state office respondents, however, said they were requiring community development as a condition of participation in the Flex Programme or CAH conversion. Five states [ii] indicated that they "strongly encouraged it," while 14 states [iii] said they required it.

It's interesting that some states that are known to be active in the community development "movement" and that invest considerable resources in these activities, are not necessarily requiring it. This would include, for example, North Dakota, Idaho and Montana. One of the explanations given is that to be a meaningful activity, community development activities must be entered into and embraced wholeheartedly and sincerely, and not as part of an institutionalized requirement.

Tennessee has employed the unique strategy of institutionalizing a community-based planning approach. Community Health Councils, which began as a grass-roots community planning effort, are a strong force in Tennessee and have been instrumental in identifying rural communities' health needs for the Flex Programme. Locally-based Community Health Councils have been turned into formal entities (staff are state employees) and are organized into eight offices for the state's 95 counties (some regional offices are responsible for up to 15 counties). Community Health Councils initiated and continue to be responsible for the formal needs assessment process called "Community Diagnosis." It was reported to us that the Department of Health funnels significant responsibility to this organization for community development. The Flex Programme has encouraged the Health Councils to become much more involved with local hospitals.

Tracking Team members found in our first round of site visits in 2000 that several hospital administrators had managed to convert their facilities to CAH status without informing their communities at all. They were quite deliberate about not wanting to "upset" their citizenry about a change that was not going to lead to any visible change in scope of services or operations. Other administrators viewed the new designation as an opportunity to fully engage business people, elected officials, the news media, patients and other providers in a discussion about the future of health care in their towns, and even celebrated the new designation as a federal recognition of the "critical" nature of their hospitals. Only five of the 30 state offices surveyed reported that they believed there were communities in their states engaging in "stealth" conversions. The Tracking Team did not encounter such conversions during our second round of site visits (2001). Florida reported that some hospitals "have come out with a big ribbon-cutting ceremony," while others view it as strictly a reimbursement strategy. In Maine, it was reported there were community meetings about the conversion decision that brought out "citizens who were worried about the services being limited," while other communities had similar meetings that no one attended. In Texas, town hall meetings are a mandatory part of the application process for every converting hospital.

Some states reported that their offices were highly involved in local community development activities. Arkansas is using the "Hometown Health Initiative" in 11 of its communities. California is helping communities conduct needs assessments, and is doing economic impact statements for three communities this summer. Florida's office has worked with 29 communities, meeting with hospital boards and staffs and local government officials, and conducting community meetings. Iowa reports working with 20 communities. Louisiana has worked with a similar number, and has organized teams to meet with county commissioners and others. Michigan offers technical assistance, and has sent state office staff into 22 communities. North Dakota's office works with communities to conduct needs assessments and strategic planning, and has visited 22 communities under the Flex Programme. Twelve of North Dakota's 14 CAHs have engaged in some form of community development, including assessments, community forums, key informant interviews, and strategic planning. Minnesota's office of rural health is very busy in communities, as is Oklahoma, Tennessee and Oregon.

One community development trainer told an audience at the 2000 National Rural Health Association conference in New Orleans that the most important requirement for a community developer is the possession of a valid driver's license. We believe the states where staff have developed active and meaningful relationships with the hospitals in their states, and who make frequent trips to visit those facilities, are the states making the most effective use of their Flex Programmes. Some state offices of rural health reported communities in their states were very enthusiastic about the Flex Programme. "Nearly all communities are positive about the CAH programme because this programme may add to the longevity of the hospitals in their areas," Hawaii reported. In Illinois, we were told, "Board members are very positive. They see the CAH programme as an opportunity. They have to make very tough decisions to keep a hospital viable." Virginia concurs: "They are very grateful for something that can save their hospital." And in Washington: "Since communities are supporting the hospital with their taxes, it's a pretty strong statement (that they want to keep them open)."

We learned in one of our site visits that West Virginia places considerable emphasis on community development when it awards grants to CAHs, although some hospitals engage in significantly more visible activities than others. Nebraska's state office encourages CAH administrators to inform their communities of conversion decisions, and has developed a "communications kit" to assist hospitals with that process. The kit is posted to the Web at http://www.nahhsnet.org/html/CAH/cah_communicat.htm. Tennessee has institutionalized a community development process by creating standing community committees, but still finds the spirit of these activities varies widely and depends largely on local leadership.

Survey of CAH Administrators

In the fall of 2000, the University of Minnesota conducted a survey of all hospital administrators whose facilities had converted to CAH status by September 1, 2000 (see description of survey in the Introduction). Questions in the survey inquired about community support for the hospital, the frequency of meetings among all the community's health care providers, and local tax support for hospitals (as an expression of local support). Our survey finds the following associations (which may not be causal):

- Community support of hospitals (both general and financial support in tax dollars) improves with frequency of provider meetings.
- Communities that support their hospitals with tax dollars have experienced lower turnover in their hospital administration.
- Hospitals with lower turnover tend to be in communities rated supportive by the administrators.

When asked "how would you characterize the community's level of support for the hospital before conversion?" 57 percent of administrators reported that support was "high," 32 percent "medium," and 12 percent "low." Only 35 percent of hospital administrators said they met monthly or more frequently with "representatives of local public health, mental health, EMS and/or other similar community-based health care providers that were not formally affiliated with the hospital." Of the administrators who responded that they met with local providers at least monthly, however, 70 percent characterized their communities as "highly supportive" of the hospitals. Only half of the administrators who met less frequently reported that their communities were highly supportive (significance: $p < 0.01$).

About half the administrators reported that they received local tax dollars to support the hospital. Two-thirds of the administrators who reported at least monthly meetings with other providers received tax support, while three-fourths of those who did not receive tax support met less frequently than monthly. We may conclude from these findings that administrators who take the time and make the effort to engage with non-hospital health care providers in the community are reaping rewards of better community support. Site visits support this conclusion. As we discuss in our chapter on hospital administration, administrator turnover is a serious problem in rural hospitals, and tends to be associated with hospital financial distress. Almost a third of the hospital administrators reported that their hospitals had more than two administrators in the past five years. However, only 25 percent of communities that support their hospitals with tax dollars experienced high turnover (defined as more than two administrators in the last five years) compared to 37 percent of communities that provided no tax support (significance: $p = 0.075$). These associations probably flow from a complex web of community culture, and it is difficult to tease out the root cause (does tax support lead to reduced turnover, or does reduced turnover lead to the stability that leads communities to support their hospitals with taxes?).

Another survey finding was that hospitals with lower administrator turnover tended to be associated with communities that were rated highly supportive by the administrators. While 62 percent of the low-turnover hospitals were in "high support" rated communities, only 46 percent of high-turnover hospitals were in "high support" communities (significance: $p = 0.079$). A conclusion we can entertain from these latter findings is that communities that support their hospitals with local tax dollars and that have general community enthusiasm regarding the hospital may enjoy lower hospital administrator turnover.

Community Site Visits

Tracking Team site visits in both of the past two years lead us to believe there are few communities where conversion is controversial. This is especially true since the 96-hour stay rule became a facility-wide average rather than a per-case requirement.

There are a few towns where citizens, staff or physicians fail to understand the true nature of the programme, in which case there may be local opposition. This has occurred, for example, in communities in some of the original states that participated in the pre-cursor Rural Primary Care Hospital (PCH) programme. In communities where facilities and opinion leaders had considered participation in the PCH programme and rejected it (for whatever reason), it seems to be more difficult to "re-visit" the conversion decision under this new Flex programme. There are also communities where physicians whipped up local opposition by characterizing the programme as a "downsizing" initiative. Nonetheless, these are rare exceptions to the general experience. A few, but not many, of the CAH conversion communities we visited are spending considerable effort on creating collaborative relationships between and among health care providers within the same town. The efforts of four of the hospitals that we visited provide interesting examples of intra-community networking. Their preliminary efforts suggest the benefits that may accrue to hospitals and communities that engage in this exercise. Providers from one New Mexico CAH routinely meet with other community providers as part of a local perinatal providers' group and a maternal and child health coalition. These committees serve as an informal case management service for low-income women in their community. A northern Michigan CAH has worked with the local county health department and the local American Indian tribes to expand women's services, including diagnostic testing. Representatives from the same hospital also serve on the local human services collaborative board with a wider variety of community agencies including public health, mental health, and domestic violence agencies. The board is charged with analyzing and addressing local coordination and service issues. A North Carolina CAH has close relationships to the local health department and supports part of the Director's salary. In addition to expanding programmes (a diabetic programme, for example) to underserved populations, the hospital has also been in a position to maintain public health services in their community in the face of state budget cuts.

A CAH in central West Virginia has partnered with the local school department to open a clinic at the school. The clinic is available to students and staff as well as their families on a sliding fee scale. No patient is turned away because of an inability to pay. The hospital is planning an additional school-based clinic in a nearby community. This clinic will be the only source of primary care in that town.

These CAH-based programmes have not only expanded services to vulnerable populations in the communities where they are located, but have also helped to identify the hospital as essential community provider. As a result, the administrators report greater community support, which has translated into the maintenance of tax support in one community and expanded private fund raising capacity in another. Three of the administrators specifically noted increased utilization of ambulatory and outpatient services resulting from their local networking efforts.

While not the highest Flex Programme priority, it does appear that a substantial amount of community development activity is associated with the programme and that this activity varies by state. State offices of rural health are involved in varying degrees with facilitating community development work in CAH conversion and non-conversion communities. There are complex interrelationships between community development, hospital success, administrator turnover, and the CAH conversion process. While not all of the community development activities we enumerate were a direct consequence of the Flex/CAH Programme, we believe the programme is directly responsible for some of them and has acted as a catalyst for many of the rest. Furthermore, we believe these types of activities are essential to the long-term viability of the CAHs.

PHYSICIAN PERCEPTIONS OF THE CRITICAL ACCESS HOSPITAL

The Flex Programme allows a variety of approaches to be implemented for the purpose of improving the rural health delivery system. As noted elsewhere in this report, states are encouraged to use programme funds to improve rural emergency medical service (EMS) and community development in addition to critical access hospital (CAH) designation. Ultimately, the success of the Flex Programme depends, in part, on the rural health care workforce, including facility administrators and the community's providers of health care. Based on discussions with administrators and a survey of physicians of CAHs conducted by Project HOPE Walsh Center for Rural Health Analysis, our impressions are that conversion has either helped or has not affected facility-physician relations. In this chapter, we examine how physicians perceive the impacts of CAH conversion, both on their own practice of medicine and on their community's health care infrastructure.

Methods

Construction of the Sampling Frame

We conducted a four-page mail survey of physicians who are currently affiliated with a CAH that has been functioning for at least one year. The sampling frame of affiliated physicians was constructed by identifying 158 CAHs of interest, and then identifying physicians who practice in each CAH's "market area." CAHs of interest were those facilities that acquired the CAH designation prior to April 2000, as we wanted to focus on facilities with the most experience as CAHs. These facilities were identified from the list maintained by the University of North Carolina. An initial list of physicians was constructed from electronic telephone listings of physicians' practices (1) with addresses having the same ZIP code as the CAH, and (2) with addresses having ZIP codes that were physically contiguous to the area defined by the CAH's ZIP code. A physician was deemed to be potentially eligible for the survey if his/her practice address was within the CAH's "market area," defined as within 15 (driving) miles of the CAH. The final step was determining the status of the physician's affiliation with the CAH. We telephoned each of the 158 eligible CAHs, and asked for a list of physicians who either treated patients at the facility or had some affiliation with the facility. Our final sampling frame contained physicians who appeared on the list provided by the CAHs *and* on our telephone list of market area physicians. Physicians who were identified by the facility as affiliated physicians, but were not on our list, were included in the final sampling frame *after* verification that the practice was located in the CAH's market area. Physicians who were on our list were *not* included in the sampling frame if they were not listed as an affiliated physician by the CAH. A total of 621 physicians were included in the final sampling frame.

Data Collection

The survey instrument was designed to obtain information on effects of conversion on the physician's practice, and physician perceptions of the effects on the facility and the community. A copy of the instrument is provided in Appendix D. A packet was mailed to each physician in the sample of affiliated physicians. The packet contained a personalized cover letter explaining the nature of the survey, the survey instrument, a business reply envelope, and an honorarium check for $20, in an attempt to maximise the response rate. A reminder postcard was mailed to surveyed physicians who had not responded after the first week. Follow-up reminder calls were placed to non-responding physicians beginning three weeks after the initial mailing. The data collection period continued for approximately eight weeks.

Estimation

Three sets of estimates based on the survey data are

reported below. First, we provide background information on the population of physicians who are affiliated with a CAH. By definition, affiliation means that the physician sees patients at the facility (although not necessarily frequently). Second, we focus on the subset of affiliated physicians who were *also* affiliated with the facility *prior to* conversion. Estimates address whether conversion to CAH status has affected the numbers of inpatients and outpatients treated by the physician and inpatient and ER outcomes.

We hypothesized that conversion would have little or no effect on inpatient volume, based on anecdotal evidence from discussions with administrators during our site visits. Several administrators indicated that any anticipated changes in service volume and service mix that might be related to conversion probably occurred prior to the actual conversion. We had no expectations concerning outpatient volume effects.

We asked physicians about perceived changes in inpatient outcomes because both positive and negative opinions have been expressed about possible consequences of conversion. Although administrators indicated that conversion should not adversely affect outcomes, several expressed concerns raised in their communities that outcomes and quality of care would deteriorate as facilities "are no longer full-service hospitals." We asked physicians about changes in ER outcomes because the Flex Programme permits the targeting of funds to EMS activities, and it was possible that CAH conversion could lead to changes in the CAH ER and/or the local EMS system.

Finally, we report estimates that describe the affiliated physician's *current* experiences with the CAH. These estimates, based on the entire sample of currently affiliated physicians, concern the nature of communication with the CAH's administration, the physician's perceptions of how conversion has affected the community, and personal satisfaction with the facility's decision to convert. We focus on whether the physician has received communication from the CAH's administration on two issues that are important in utilisation management - the types of treatment that the CAH will offer to inpatients and inpatient length of stay. We do not have any hypotheses about these factors, as the urgency of utilisation management efforts may have been weakened when the 96-hour rule was changed from a per-stay limit to an average. Most facilities that were candidates for conversion had a length of stay less than 96 hours before conversion. We hypothesize that the Flex Programme has strengthened the community's medical infrastructure, and expect to see this expressed by affiliated physicians.

Estimates presented below are primarily of a descriptive nature. We report means of continuous variables and percents for categorical data. Standard errors and the number of respondents are also provided, should the reader desire to calculate selected confidence intervals and conduct tests of statistical significance.

Findings

Characteristics of Affiliated Physicians

A total of 471 physicians completed the mail survey, resulting in a response rate of about 76 percent. A subset of 430 respondents, who currently see inpatients at the CAH in their market area, is the group of interest in this analysis. Of these physicians, 179 (42%) characterize themselves as staff physicians employed by the CAH, and 251 (58%) are members of independent practices who see inpatients at the CAH (Table 1).

TABLE 1

Characteristics of Physicians Affiliated with a Critical Access Hospital

	Number of Respondents	*Mean or Percent (Standard Error)*
Current Relationship with CAH:		
Staff Physician	179	41.6% (2.4)
Independent Practice	251	58.4% (2.4)
Specialty:		
General/Family Practice	263	61.3% (2.4)
Medicine Specialties	114	26.6% (2.1)
Surgical Specialties	17	8.2% (1.3)
Other	35	4.0% (0.9)
Time in practice since medical school, in years	428	18.9 (0.5)
Years of practice in community	424	10.2 (0.5)
Total hours worked, preceding week, all practices and settings	427	58.9 (0.9)
Percent of time worked, preceding week, in CAH community only	422	86.1 (1.4)
Number of CAH inpatients admitted during past month	406	11.0 (0.5)

Source: Walsh Center Survey of Physicians Affiliated with a CAH, 2001.

Sixty-one percent of physicians with a CAH affiliation (also to be referred to as "CAH-affiliates" below) are general or family practitioners. About 88 percent of affiliates specify general or family practice or a medical specialty as their primary specialty. The remaining 12 percent of CAH-affiliated physicians are surgical specialists (8%) and other specialists (4%). Although the average CAH-affiliated physician has been practicing for about 19 years since completing medical school training, the amount of time the physician has practiced in the community served by the CAH is considerably less — 10 years. The distribution of time in the community, however, is very skewed. About one-half of CAH-affiliates have practiced in their communities for five years or less; 17 percent have practicing in their current community for more than 20 years.

The work week of the average CAH-affiliate is lengthy. The average CAH-affiliate worked 59 hours during the week prior to the survey, and 25 percent of respondents reported working in excess of 70 hours during that week. Much of the affiliate's work time is in the CAH community. The average CAH-affiliate spent 86 percent of his/her work time in the community during the week prior to the survey, and only 20 percent of respondents spent less than 80 percent of their work hours in the community.

There is considerable variation in the number of patients admitted to the CAH by CAH-affiliates. The mean number of admissions during the previous month was 11. About 47 percent had fewer than 10 admissions, while 18 percent reported 20 or more.

Impacts of Conversion

Of the 430 physician respondents who are currently affiliated with a CAH, 375 (87%) also treated patients at the facility prior to conversion. The survey was designed to obtain several measures of the extent to which conversion has affected these physicians' practice of medicine.

Patient Volume. Most physicians (80%) reported no change in the number of inpatients treated at the CAH, or in the number of outpatients treated at either the CAH and in their office (79%) as a result of the conversion (Table 2). About 16 percent reported a change in inpatient volume, with two-thirds of those reporting a change (11% overall) reporting a decrease in inpatient volume. The opposite effect, however, was observed among the 15 percent of physicians reporting a change in outpatient volume. Among these physicians, most (13% overall) reported that conversion increased outpatient volume. We cannot determine whether this increase resulted from changes in outpatient services provided at the CAH or at the physician's office.

TABLE 2

Impacts of Conversion on Patient Volume

Percent Reporting Volume Effect*

Patient Type	*Increase*	*No Change*	*Decrease*	*Don't Know*
Inpatients at CAH (N=370)	4.9 (1.1)	80.0 (2.1)	10.8 (1.6)	4.3 (1.1)
All Outpatients (N=371)	13.2 (1.8)	79.2 (2.1)	1.9 (0.7)	5.7 (1.2)

Notes: *Standard error in parentheses.
Source: Walsh Center Survey of Physicians Affiliated with a CAH, 2001.

Communication with the CAH Administration

Most physicians had not recently received information from the CAH administration that was targeted at limiting treatment of patients with certain conditions or affecting change in inpatient length of stay. Only 19 percent of physicians received information concerning *limits on treatments*. Among recipients, this information was not well received. Sixty-four percent of those physicians who received this information viewed it as compromising their practice, whereas only 17 percent found the information beneficial.

Patient Outcomes. A key issue is whether conversion has affected outcomes of patients using the CAH and ER, given the Flex Program's potential impacts on inpatient stays and the local EMS system. Most (76% overall, and 85% of those with an opinion) reported no impact on inpatient outcomes, and 72 percent reported no impact on outcomes among patients using the ER (Table 3). Among those reporting a change in outcomes, most reported improved outcomes in each setting. The number of physicians reporting improved inpatient outcomes exceeded the number reporting worsened outcomes by a factor of 3.8 for inpatients and 6.8 for ER patients.

TABLE 3

Impacts of Conversion on Outcomes

Percent Reporting Outcome Effect*

Patient Type	*Improved*	*No Change*	*Worsened*	*Don't Know*
Inpatients at CAH (N=370)	10.3 (1.6)	76.2 (2.2)	2.7 (0.8)	10.8 (1.6)
Patients using ER (N=371)	10.8 (1.6)	72.2 (2.3)	1.6 (0.7)	15.4 (1.9)

Notes: *Standard error in parentheses.

Source: Walsh Center Survey of Physicians Affiliated with a CAH, 2001.

Forty percent of physicians received information targeted at changing *inpatient length of stay*, and as expected, the communication encouraged length of stay reduction for most of these physicians - 36 percent overall, or 90 percent of the 40 percent receiving length of stay information. As with communication concerning changes in treatment of patients with certain conditions, communication concerning changes in length of stay was viewed negatively: 78 percent of length of stay information recipients thought this information compromised their practices, and only 10 percent found it to be beneficial to their practices.

Physician Perceptions of Community Views and Infrastructure Impacts

Although conversion seems not to have had significant impacts on the volumes of inpatients and outpatients, nor on changes in conditions treated in the facility, physicians viewed conversion as having effects on the facility's image in the community and on the community's health care infrastructure. Although most physicians believed that conversion had not changed community views on quality of care at the facility (68%), 59 percent of those who thought community perceptions had changed (18% overall) believed that community members perceived that quality of care improved.

Approximately six of 10 respondents indicated that conversion has had no effect on the attractiveness of the community as a desirable place for them to practice. Of the 40 percent who indicated that conversion affected the attractiveness of the community for their practice, more physicians indicated the effect was beneficial than negative, by a factor of over two to one - 27 percent versus 12 percent.

A related issue is whether physicians believe that conversion has improved the community's ability to attract new physicians. Nineteen percent indicated that conversion improved the community's ability to attract physicians, whereas 8 percent indicated that community attractiveness to other physicians had worsened. Forty-two percent of physicians believed that conversion had no impact, and 31 percent were not aware of changes in the community's attractiveness from the perspective of other physicians.

Support for the conversion's positive effect on the stability of the community's infrastructure was considerably stronger than physician views on whether the conversion affected the perception of the community as a place to practice for him/herself and for others. Forty-seven percent indicated that infrastructure stability was enhanced by conversion, while only seven percent indicated that conversion has weakened the community's health care infrastructure.

Physician Support for Conversion

Overall support by physicians for conversion was very positive. Nearly 70 percent were supportive of conversion, and only 8 percent opposed or strongly opposed conversion. Other physicians were neutral, neither expressing support nor opposition.

Discussion

Perhaps the most important conclusion from this analysis is that physicians are very supportive of the facility's decision to become a CAH. This conclusion is reassuring, as it is consistent with claims by the typical CAH administrator, during Tracking Team site visits, that the medical staff is supportive of conversion once the conversion process is explained. We are not able to fully account for the reasons for physician support. Survey results suggest that some support stems from perceived effects of the CAH on the stability of the community's health care infrastructure. However, support does not appear to stem directly from perceived conversion effects on the attractiveness of the community as a place to practice or in attracting other physicians. We suspect that some of the advantages of conversion are only a subset of the factors that determine whether the community is an attractive place to practice medicine. Project HOPE researchers are continuing to study the nature of physician support for conversion.

A second conclusion from this analysis is that conversion *per se* does not appear to have dramatically affected the day-to-day practice of medicine by physicians who affiliate with a CAH. Most physicians reported no changes in the volumes of inpatients and outpatients, nor did most physicians report perceived changes in inpatient outcomes and outcomes of ER patients that could be attributed to conversion. Again, the lack of immediate effects of conversion on inpatient volume is consistent with our in-the-field discussions with CAH administrators. Why most physicians *who reported outcome effects* of conversion reported positive effects cannot be determined from the survey data. One hypothesis, however, is that physicians are aware of efforts by CAH administration, observed during the Tracking Team's site visits, to implement quality improvements. At the same time, conversion has not been painless for physicians. Some-albeit a small number-indicated that their practices were adversely affected by challenges from CAH administration to limit treatment of certain types of conditions at the CAH (12% of CAH-affiliates), and a larger number reported adverse effects of challenges by CAH administration to reduce inpatient length of stay (28%).

Finally, it is important to emphasize that results from this survey describe physicians *who are affiliated with CAHs*. Clearly, this is an important set of providers in rural communities that have received funds from the Flex Programme. We believe that monitoring of affiliate physicians in the future is important, as some of the effects of conversion may become apparent only as time passes. But it is also important to recognize that other physician providers practice in communities served by CAHs. In fact, we estimate that there are about as many non-affiliates as affiliate physicians who serve CAH communities. We have not studied this important group of providers - a group that is not likely to be as supportive of the CAH concept and of the Flex Programme. Hence, our results should be interpreted with caution and with the understanding that study of the reactions of non-affiliated providers to the Flex Programme is warranted.

4

Public Health Authority & Public Hospital Administration

Public Health Authority and Responsibility

A naturopathic doctor is a licensed doctor and has the same authority and responsibility as other licensed doctors regarding public health laws, reportable disease and conditions, communicable disease control and prevention, recording of vital statistics, health and physical examinations and local boards of health, except that this authority is limited to activity consistent with the scope of practice authorized by this chapter.

CASE STUDY: SAN FRANCISCO HEALTH AUTHORITY

Establishment

Pursuant to the authority granted to the City and County of San Francisco by Welfare and Institutions Code Section 14087.36 (hereafter, "Section 14087.36"), there is hereby established the San Francisco Health Authority as a public entity separate and distinct from the City and County of San Francisco.

Purpose

The San Francisco Health Authority recognizes that Medi-Cal beneficiaries have traditionally faced a significant lack of access to health care and have been dependent upon traditional, safety net, and other concerned providers for needed health care services. The City and private providers of health care and other interested parties have collaborated in the development of a managed care plan and the San Francisco Health Authority is established as the result of this collaborative effort. The Board of Supervisors has determined to establish the Health Authority as the Local Initiative under the Medi-Cal program. The Board of Supervisors has determined that it is in the public interest to establish the Health Authority to create an efficient, integrated health care delivery system in order to provide, as contracted by the California State Department of Health Services with the Authority, access to comprehensive health care services for Medi-Cal beneficiaries and such other persons as the Health Authority deems appropriate; to provide quality care that is compassionate, respectful and culturally and linguistically appropriate; and to ensure preservation of the safety net.

Powers and Responsibilities

(a) The San Francisco Health Authority shall be the local initiative component of the Medi-Cal state plan pursuant to regulations adopted by the State Department of Health Services.

(b) The Health Authority may undertake all actions and perform all functions authorized by Section 14087.36 or otherwise permitted by law. In addition, the Health Authority may apply for and obtain licensure as a health care service plan under Health and Safety Code Section 1340 et seq. and, once so licensed, may engage in all activities permitted of a health care service plan.

(c) The Health Authority may enter into contracts to provide or arrange for health care services for persons eligible to receive benefits under the Medi-Cal program and to other individuals, including, but not limited to, those covered under Title 42 of the United State Code, individuals employed by public agencies and private businesses, and uninsured or indigent individuals.

(d) The Health Authority shall have all the rights, powers, duties, privileges, immunities, and obligations provided pursuant to Section 14087.36.

(e) Members of the governing body of the Health Authority shall not be compensated for their service on the governing body, but may be reimbursed for authorized expenses under procedures established by the governing body.

(f) The Health Authority may adopt rules and regulations governing the operation and procedures of the governing body and the Authority, provided that such rules and regulations are not in conflict with the provisions of Section 14087.36.

Governing Body

(a) The governing body of the Health Authority shall consist of 19 members who shall have the qualifications required by Section 14087.36. The Board of Supervisors shall, by resolution, appoint 14 persons pursuant to the nomination procedure set forth in Section 14087.36. The Mayor shall appoint a person to serve at the pleasure of the Mayor. The Director of Public Health, the Director of Mental Health, and the Chancellor of the University of California at San Francisco shall each serve as a member or appoint a designee to serve at his or her pleasure. The Health Commission shall appoint a person to serve at its pleasure. Appointments and changes in appointment, other than those of the Board of Supervisors, shall be made by filing written notice with the Clerk of the Board of Supervisors.

(b) All members of the governing body shall be voting members except the member appointed by the San Francisco Health Commission.

(c) The initial members appointed by the Board of Supervisors shall be, to the extent those individuals meet the qualifications required by Section 14087.36(k) and are willing to serve, those persons serving as members of the San Francisco Managed Care Steering Committee.

(d) The term of office for each member appointed by the Board of Supervisors shall be three years, commencing at 12:00 noon, on the 15th day of January in the year 1995; provided that at the initial meeting of the governing body the members appointed by the Board of Supervisors shall draw lots to determine seven members whose initial terms of office shall be for two years; and provided further that the person appointed pursuant to Section 14087.36(k)(1)(A) as a member or representative of the Board of Supervisors shall serve at the pleasure of the Board.

(e) For purposes of Government Code Section 87103, the members of the governing body are appointed to represent and further the interests of the specific health care providers and other interests specified in Section 14087.36(k) and (q).

(f) The filling of vacant positions, the rights of members whose terms have expired, voting procedures, the selection of the chair, the establishment of committees, and the procedure for changing the composition of the governing body and the appointment of members shall be as set forth in Section 14087.36.

(g) A member of the governing body may be removed from office by the Board of Supervisors by resolution, but only upon the recommendation of the Health Authority and for the reasons specified in Section 14087.36.

(h) A member of the governing body may resign from office by submitting a written notice of resignation to the Health Authority. The Health Authority shall notify the Clerk of the Board of Supervisors of the resignation within five days.

(i) Upon approval of this ordinance, the Clerk of the Board shall schedule a hearing before an appropriate committee of the Board for consideration of the appointment of members to the governing body of the Health Authority. The Clerk shall provide notice of the hearing to persons and entities with the authority to nominate and to other interested parties.

(j) The Health Authority shall notify the Board of Supervisors four months prior to the expiration of any term of office of a member of the governing body. The Clerk shall promptly notify the entity with the authority to nominate a person for the position that a nomination is required and must be submitted within 30 days. Upon receipt of the nomination, the Clerk shall schedule a hearing before an appropriate committee of the Board for consideration of the appointment. If a position on the governing body becomes vacant, the Health Authority shall promptly notify the Clerk, who shall notify the nominating authority for the vacant position and, upon receipt of the nomination, schedule a hearing before the appropriate committee of the Board for consideration of an appointment to fill the vacant position.

Required Insurance

The Risk Manager of the City and County shall determine the type and amount of insurance that is reasonably necessary to enable the Health Authority to provide for the defense and indemnification of employees of the Health Authority who are employees of the City and County of San Francisco, as required by Section 14087.36(d)(1)(A). The Health

Authority shall provide insurance of the amount and type, and subject to such terms and conditions, as may be required by the Risk Manager, including any changes in that determination that may be appropriate for reasons that the Risk Manager shall provide in writing.

When Constituted

The Health Authority may take official action once a majority of the voting members of the governing body have been appointed.

TRANSITION IN A PUBLIC HOSPITAL ADMINISTRATION: A CASE STUDY FROM SOWETO

This chapter investigates the impact of the triple transition on the workplace in South Africa's biggest hospital, Chris Hani Baragwanath Hospital in Soweto. It explores the paralysis and internal decomposition of the workplace regime as it is crushed between two forces – budget cutbacks and the concomitant staff shortages on the one hand, and the breakdown of managerial structures and disciplinary relations on the other. Lacking robust and effective managerial structures and systems, the institution is subject to a slow unravelling of workplace relations and practices, and a deterioration in the quality of bothhealth care and working life. The chapter also documents a trade union initiative to reconstruct workplace order on a new basis.

Public service workplaces have been relatively invisible in the evolution of progressiveindustrial sociology research in South Africa, with its focus on private-sector manufacturing and mining. This study of the health sector constitutes a first step towards attempting tounderstand the specific character of the workplace regime in the public service and to facilitate a comparison with the changing workplace regime in industry. What was thecharacter of the apartheid workplace regime in the public service, specifically in hospitals? In what ways did it resemble or differ from the apartheid workplace regime in the private sector (Von Holdt 2003b)? Has it been affected by the transition in similar ways? To what extent is the nature of workplace order subject to contestation? Is a distinct post-apartheid workplace regime emerging?

This Study

The research for this study developed out of a trade union initiative for the transformation of Chris Hani Baragwanath Hospital into a 'People's Hospital' which would improve the quality of health-care service as well as the quality of working life for union members. In 2000, officials of the National Education Health and Allied Workers Union (NEHAWU) approached the National Labour and Economic Development Institute (NALEDI)2to assistwith this project. After a series of workshops and discussions with NEHAWU shop stewards, NALEDI drew up an initial report on behalf of the union with broad proposals for change (NEHAWU 2001). This was presented to management, the hospital Board and the other trade unions at the institution, and finally adopted as a framework document by all stakeholders at the beginning of 2002 (Towards a People's Hospital 2002). The Surgical Department was chosen as a pilot project for the implementation of change, and NALEDI was commissionedto undertake in-depth research into the functioning of this department. Interviews and focus groups were arranged with all levels of staff, from cleaners to doctors, and proposals for change were designed based on the results. The research and proposals were then presented to the trade unions and management at a Transformation Forum – itself established as an element of the stakeholder agreement (NALEDI 2002). –There, agreement was reached that the proposals would be implemented as a pilot project for change in the Surgical Department.The process of creating the conditions for implementation began early in 2003.

This study is based on the research into shop stewards' views undertaken for the initial report in 2000, the interviews and focus groups conducted for the research into the SurgicalDepartment in 2002, and the research information gathered through a process of participantobservation. NALEDI was a participant in trade union, shop steward and managementmeetings by virtue of its role as adviser in the transformation project – a role which alsoentailed numerous information-rich informal discussions with all parties. The authors of this chapter are NALEDI researchers. The researchers' location in the institution as activeprotagonists – as advocates for a more participatory, democratic and co-operative workplace environment – obviously colours the research as well as the arguments put forward in this chapter; indeed, the substance of the chapter constitutes an argument for specific policychanges in order to reconstruct the institution. However, both the research findings and the arguments for change have been tested by robust exchanges within the institution as well as with senior officials in the national and Gauteng departments of health, as well as in the arduous process of attempting to implement change.Indeed, there is nothing like the practiceof grappling with the challenges and difficulties of institutional change for generating rich knowledge about the workings of institutional structures and practices.

The Hospital

Baragwanath Hospital – the name of assassinated Communist leader Chris Hani wasadded in 1997 to signify the reorientation of the hospital in the new democratic era – was established as a military hospital with 1 500 beds during World War II, and later convertedinto a civilian hospital for the African residents of the Witwatersrand. After the war, the African section of Johannesburg General Hospital, consisting of 480 beds, was transferred to Baragwanath. When Soweto was established around the site of Baragwanath by the apartheid government during the 1950s, the hospital became the main health-care facility serving the residents of the vast African township. Indeed, it was something of a showcase project for successive white governments to demonstrate that they did indeed care for blacks.

By the 1990s the hospital had grown to accommodate over 3 000 beds (reputedly the biggest in the world), although by the end of the decade only 2 600 were in use because offinancial constraints. Chris Hani Baragwanath is a vast institution, consisting of 429 buildings spread out over extensive grounds. Most of the wards are long, low, barrack-like structures. In 2003 there were some 5 000 people working there, including 2 000 nurses and 600 doctors. It is one of four tertiary hospitals – that is, a specialist hospital with links to an academic teaching and research institution – in Gauteng province, and is the site for the greater part of the teaching and clinical research of the University of the Witwatersrand medical faculty(www.chrishanibaragwanathhospital.co.za).

The Department of General Surgery consists of eight wards with a total of some 250 beds. Specialist surgical departments add another eight wards. The staff complement for the surgical departments consists of roughly 200 nurses, 40 ward attendants, 25 clerks and 30 cleaners. There are 80 doctors in the General Surgical Department. The wards are big – most have 32 beds, while the biggest has 60-odd beds – and are arranged on either side of a long sloping corridor, the Surgical Corridor. The busiest ward is the Surgical Admissions Ward, which admits patients from

Casualty. From here patients are distributed to the male and female wards. In the wards, patients are prepared for surgery, and post-trauma and post-operative recovery is managed.

The nursing staff consist of a distinctive hierarchy. At the bottom are the ward attendants who carry out non-nursing duties – operating the kitchen (warming and dishing up food, making and serving tea), cleaning lockers, working in the sluice room, packing the clean linen distributed from the laundry and collecting soiled linen for return to the laundry. Nursing auxiliaries, who have a year of practical and theoretical training, wash patients, make beds, record patients' vital data, distribute certain levels of medication, apply dressings, and escortpatients to other parts of the hospital or to other hospitals. Staff nurses, with an additional year of training, have additional tasks – accompanying ward rounds, writing a daily patient report, administering medication up to schedule-five drugs, preparing patients for theatre, and so on.

Professional nurses have completed a four-year training programme and are accountable for health care. They manage the other nursing staff, administer scheduled drugs, and can apply ventilation and resuscitation equipment. They also have a range of administrative and managerial tasks such as planning staff allocations and ordering stock. After three years ofpractical work, professional nurses are generally promoted to become senior professional nurses, and after a further three years to chief professional nurses (CPN).

Currently, most wards are expected to have four professional nurses, two auxiliary nurses and two ward attendants on day shift, each working four days on and four days off per week. This means that on six days per week there are half this number actually on duty. Night shiftsare generally expected to operate with a smaller number of staff – a professional nurse and an auxiliary nurse, with a ward attendant shared between two wards.

Each ward also has a number of support workers – one or two cleaners managed by a supervisor and foreman located in offices far from the wards, and a ward clerk managed by a supervisor in the corridor outside the ward. The ward is managed by the most senior chief professional nurse on duty on each shift. She is accountable to the corridor supervisors or matrons, who are stationed in an office in the Surgical Corridor, and each of whom oversees four wards. The corridor supervisors in turn are managed by a nursing assistant director for the surgical wards, stationed in the administration block. The surgeons are managed by the surgical chief clinician, and apart from actually conducting operations they prescribe the clinical dimension of health care on ward rounds and on individual visits to their patients.

An Overview of the Democratic Transition and Change at the Hospital

First, a word of caution: the primary purpose of this study was to understand the currentdynamics of workplace order and disorder, rather than to probe the nature of workplace practices before the democratic breakthrough (1990-94). The precise nature of control and authority and the dynamics of compliance and resistance during the period of apartheid require further research. Nonetheless, certain characteristics can be gleaned from interviewsand conversations with those who have worked at the hospital for many years. One aspect isworth remarking on – many, if not all, interviewees expressed a certain nostalgia for the timewhen Baragwanath functioned effectively as a hospital, a time when supervisors knew how to supervise and discipline was discipline.

Because Baragwanath hospital was a 'black' hospital, the transition to democracy did not imply a reorientation to serve a new community, as it did for 'white' hospitals such as the Johannesburg General Hospital. The impact of the transition was felt far more in terms of internal institutional relations and dynamics – changes in the racial division of labour, the recognition of trade unions, and changing attitudes towards and practices of discipline.

As in the private sector, the institution was characterised by a rigid racial division of labour during the period of apartheid. During the 1980s virtually the entire senior and middlemanagement layers were white, including clinical, administrative and financial management. Most doctors and paramedical professional staff – radiologists, physiotherapists, and so on – were also white. Most nursing and clerical staff, and all support workers such as cleaners, porters, ward attendants and security guards, were black. What distinguished the workplace regime at Baragwanath, as a hospital serving black communities, from workplaces in the private sector was that the biggest contingent of professional workers, the nursing staff, was almost entirely black. This constituted a highly skilled group, including significantsupervisory layers.

Apart from the somewhat distinctive racial division of labour, the apartheid workplace regime at Baragwanath was characterised by a hierarchical and disciplinarian managerial style, and a strict, even despotic, disciplinary regime for black workers. By the end of the 1980s the industrial relations regime in the public service still resembled the classical apartheid workplace regime as it had existed in the private sector at the beginning of the 1970s, before the resurgence of black trade unionism and the labour reforms of 1980. Public service workers had no trade union, collective bargaining or dispute resolution rights. The Labour

Relations Act (1981) specifically excluded public service employees. White public service trade unions engaged in practices of consultation with a white government which was sympathetic to their concerns (Nyembe 1992). Black public service workers had little job security and no recourse against unfair dismissals. Public service institutions such as Baragwanath Hospital were characterised by personnel administration departments rather than industrial relations or labour relations functions, mirroring the situation in industry at the beginning of the 1970s.

In the late 1980s, trade union organisation of black workers in the public service was inits infancy. NEHAWU was launched in 1987 as an affiliate of the Congress of South African Trade Unions (COSATU), but in 1988 had only 6 000 members drawn mostly from supportworkers in the health sector (Baskin 1991: 217, 282). The situation among nurses was somewhat different. All nurses were obliged to belong to the South African NursingAssociation (SANA), a statutory organisation dominated by white nurses and bureaucrats. With its strong professional and elitist ideology, and its hostility towards any form of trade unionism for nurses, SANA served more as an institution for the control of black nurses thana vehicle for negotiating workplace conditions and practices (Gwagwa and Webber 1995). Indeed, nursing had 'long been one of the few paths for training and better paid employmentopen to African women', and many nurses, particularly the older generation, internalised the hierarchical, disciplinarian and status-driven values of the profession. (Keet 1992: 51; see also Gwagwa and Webber 1995) Thus, in contrast to industry, black trade unionism in the public service, and specifically in the health sector, only flourished after 1990 – that is, it was more a phenomenon of the transition than of the anti-apartheid struggle.

By the time this study was undertaken (2001-4) much of this had changed. Public serviceworkers had full collective bargaining and organisational rights regulated by the Labour Relations Act (1995). NEHAWU had become the second-biggest affiliate of COSATU, and there were several other public service unions affiliated to the National Council of Trade Unions and the Federation of Trade Unions of South Africa. SANA had been disbanded and absorbed into the Democratic Nurses Organisation of South Africa (DENOSA), which affiliated to COSATU in 2003 and competes with other health sector unions for nurses'membership.

In the institution itself, white senior management had been largely replaced by black managers (two out of three directors, both senior clinical executives, and three out of five deputy directors), although there remained a larger contingent of white middle managers, particularly in administrative, financial and personnel functions. Relations between management and the four recognised trade unions – NEHAWU, DENOSA, the Hospital and Other Services Personnel of South Africa (HOSPERSA), and the National Union of Public Service Workers (NUPSW) – were characterised by regular consultative meetings and elaborate disciplinary procedures. However, as will be shown below, these changes had ushered in a process of decomposition of workplace order, rather than the formation of a new post-apartheid workplace order.

Dysfunctional Management

All staff expressed extreme frustration at what can only be called a general managerial failure at the institution. While for most staff this was most immediately apparent in the failure of supervisors and managers to exert disciplinary control – discussed below – manysaw this as simply one aspect of a broader managerial vacuum in the institution.

This was articulated most forcefully by a group of CPNs with years of accumulated experience between them:

> We are doormats for everybody. We are running this hospital for the hospital's management. When we go to meetings with our supervisors we complain about the shortage of staff, the linen, the cleaners. They tell us, "Try your best!" They come with no solutions. It is a waste of time, problems remain unresolved. Who do we cry to? We never see the managers.

A group of nursing auxiliaries endorsed this:

> Problems like staff shortage, low morale, discipline, the resignation of nurses, are not dealt with The matrons are from the wards, but as soon as they go into their offices it is as if they are in a totally different world.

There are several reasons for this – the silo system of management, an administrative and authoritarian managerial culture, and a straightforward lack of managerial capacity.

The silo system refers to the traditional health-care structure of management in which different occupational categories are managed in parallel but separate lines of managerialauthority. Thus the nursing line of authority extends all the way up from the wards to the nursing director, while the clinical line of authority extends from the doctors up to the clinical director, and the support workers are managed by a branched logistics line of authority whichculminates with the Human Resources and Logistics director. This means that no singlemanager has accountability for the effective functioning of a specified operational area suchas a ward or the Surgical Department as a whole, or the authority to manage it. Effectively,virtually every level of supervisor and management is disempowered.

The chief clinician described his frustration and his inability to implement new working practices which required the co-operation of the nursing management. Nurses complained that doctors arranged ward rounds at the busiest times of the day, when understaffed nurses were battling to complete their tasks; doctors complained that nurses failed to accompany them on ward rounds. Nurses and doctors both complained about the behaviour of cleaners and clerks, and their inability to get any response from their supervisors. Underlying such problems wasthe elusive nature of authority divided between different silos and without clear lines of accountability between them.

Instead of an integrated operational management, the fragmentation of managerialstructures into silos generates an administrative, hierarchical and authoritarian managerial culture. Managers and staff are acutely aware of status, hierarchy and the demarcations thatdefine the limits to the authority of themselves and others. They tend to focus on paperwork, administering rules, regulations and personnel, rather than managing operations, people orstrategies. Managers are isolated in the nine-floor administration block, and according to staff are seldom seen at the sites of health-care delivery. We came across several examples of 'management by memo' – managers circulating memoranda announcing decisions that were unworkable in the wards or that generated all kinds of new problems and tensions.

To the general hierarchical and authoritarian characteristics of this kind of bureaucraticculture must be added the specifically hierarchical, status-conscious and disciplinarian culture of the nursing profession (Gwagwa and Webber 1995). When we met a group of nursingauxiliaries they made a point of refusing to give us their names:

> We go to meetings and raise issues, and then they write

> our names down. We are ruled autocratically. We cannot make suggestions – they will kill you. It is like this even if there are unions.

The Assistant Director for nursing unwittingly reinforced their complaint when she said, 'The nursing auxiliaries are not a happy group. They cannot understand, they argue. I sometimes feel I should call in Security'.

The chief professional nurses responsible for running wards articulated the samecomplaint: 'The problem is that we who are in the working situation are never consulted. There is no consultation by management; to consult with us would show that they honour us'.4We came across numerous incidents of this type throughout the institution. The dysfunctional management structures and practices that characterise Chris Hani Baragwanath Hospital give rise to poor decision making with all kinds of unintended consequences, aggravating workplace inefficiency, conflict and frustration. Finally, there is the problem of management capacity. A 2003 organogram of the management structure on the hospital's web site indicates that thirteen out of 30 managementpositions were vacant. Even if they were filled, the 'management resources and expertise' would be 'less than adequate' for managing such a large and complex institution, with the result that the institution lacked a strategic plan, according to a consultant report commissioned by NALEDI (Tapson and Baker 2002: 3, 16). The same report found that the human resources (HR) function was 'under resourced, poorly structured and is focused on administration as opposed to service'. The HR director was also responsible for information technology (IT) and logistics – that is, the entire support workers silo, including the laundry, the kitchens, security, and so on. His deputy director was essentially a payroll administrator. Staffing levels had been reduced from 84 to 47 over the previous decade, and their main function was payroll and personnel administration. There was to all intents and purposes no proactive labour relations or human resources development function, no skills training for non-professional staff, no career development, career paths or functioning skills development plan, and no internal communications capacity. In short, the institution lacked a human resources strategy or the capacity to develop one.

Although the NALEDI investigation did not examine financial management in any detail, it is clear that the institution lacks financial management capacity and systems. The silostructures of management and the absence of financial systems produces a very low level of financial control, with concomitant high levels of wastage, theft and corruption. Likewise, there are no quality control systems at the hospital. In the surgical wards quality control would entail monitoring patient recovery rates, wound sepsis rates and similar indicators of the effectiveness of health-care management, so that trends could be established and health-care strategies implemented improve results. In the absence of clear accountabilities and systems, such monitoring cannot take place.

The lack of management capacity is exacerbated by the centralisation of control over many aspects of hospital functioning in the hands of the provincial health department. Thereis some controversy and a great deal of tension over this issue, but it is clear that there are very significant constraints on the scope for the hospital management to take full accountability or adopt innovative strategies. The result is 'frustration and justifiable feelings of disempowerment' so that it 'is not surprising that the capacity to promote transformation and reorganisation is largely absent' (Tapson and Baker 2002: 3).

Budget Cuts and Staff Shortages

There has been a substantial reduction in tertiary hospital budgets over the decade of democratic transformation in South Africa. This is not directly or only because of the macro-economic orthodoxy with its attendant fiscal discipline adopted as policy by the ANC government in 1996.—Indeed, the overall budget for health has remained fairly constant in financial terms over this period. More directly, it is due to a shifting emphasis within the health budget which has redistributed resources from tertiary-level to primary-level health care, and from well-resourced provinces to the poorer and more rural provinces. Nonetheless, the resulting fiscal discipline, which has been internalised by government in the form of an outer limit on the total government budget of 24 percent of GDP, does impose constraints on the resources available for health-care transformation. This general trend probably provides an explanation for the failure to address the budgetdiscrepancies that have their origins in the apartheid structure of the health services. Black hospitals were significantly under-funded in comparison to white hospitals. Chris Hani Baragwanath Hospital still suffers from this legacy. Thus, it fares worse on all measures in comparison with the formerly white Johannesburg General Hospital. While the former has almost two and a half times the beds of the latter, its expenditure is only 14 per cent more. This translates into personnel expenditure per bed, personnel expenditure per patient day, and total expenditure per bed that are 34 per cent, 70 per cent and 58 per cent, respectively, of thecomparable expenditures at the formerly white hospital. (Department of Health 2003b) The shortage of funds has placed enormous pressure on all aspects of Chris Hani Baragwanath operations. Over 1 000 of the 3 000 nursing posts specified by the 'staffing establishment' for the institution are vacant because of insufficient funding

– a staff shortageof some 30 per cent.(In comparison, both Johannesburg General and Cape Town's GrooteSchuur have nursing staff shortages of 10 per cent.) Similar reductions seem to hold for othercategories such as ward attendants and cleaners.

According to the chief surgical clinician the nursing shortage amounts to a 'crisis'. Anursing auxiliary described what this meant for his working day:

> I am the Atlas carrying the ward. I must skip my tea. I have to jump, to rush time. I must stop washing and serve tea. If there are no ward attendants I must go and make tea myself. There is no point in washing the patient and giving medications, but failing to feed him. Again, how can you leave a sick person in a wet bed, and go for lunch? In our training we were taught that you cannot wash the patient alone, but must always be two. Patients require regular turnings, and again, according to the rules, there should be two nurses to do this. At present we washalone, we turn alone, we make beds alone, irrespective of how obese or how ill the patients are.

The CPNs described their day in similar terms:

> You do not have linen today; you must phone the laundry. The dietician wants informationabout certain patients. Then a relative of the patient phones; there is no clerk to take the call and she wants the sister, so you have to deal with it. Then a doctor arrives and wants me. The supervisor of the cleaners does not respond to a complaint, so you end up sweeping the ward.If you do not have a ward attendant you must also go to the kitchen. The injections and medications are waiting. There is a patient to prepare for surgery. Then there are the reports and other paperwork. Where do you find time? At the end of the day your head is so big . . .

The result is that they have to 'prioritise ruthlessly – those being prepared for theatre, and then the critically ill and very ill. The others must just wait'. Sometimes nurses just 'top and tail' patients instead of giving them a full wash. Forfeiting tea and lunch, working overtime, working extra weekends – the workload and stress are 'unbearable'. Nurses respond to thestress by avoiding work – through resigning, coming late or absenteeism – by becoming irritable, aggressive and uncaring at work, and in some cases turning to alcohol.

The workload and stress have exacerbated relations between the different occupational categories in the wards as workers, overwhelmed by their own tasks, refuse to assist others. The result, according to the chief clinician, is 'work fragmentation'. 'The focus is not service to the patient,' he said; 'It's "I do my job, you do yours".This attitude has emerged in response to staff shortages. It was the impact of budget cuts'. The CPNs agreed. During a focus group they said, '... posts were frozen; the most important change is the shortage in staffing levels'.

A further consequence of short staffing is daily staffing crises, as the absence of a nurse or cleaner through illness or leave necessitates reshuffling staff from other hard-pressed wards. The constant reshuffling of staff prevents the building of stable working relations and creates new conflicts. The shift patterns for night staff entail regular overtime, but because of financial constraints management has issued instructions that this overtime will not be paid; instead, staff can take an equivalent amount of time off when they return to day shift. However, the staff shortages on day shift prevent this, with the result that staff haveaccumulated unmanageable amounts of overtime. The shortage of managers, itself related to financial constraints, in turn constrains the ability of management to approach these and other problems in a strategic manner.

Discipline

All staff, from cleaners to doctors, complain that a significant minority of workers in every category are ill-disciplined, lazy, absent without cause, drink at work, or are guilty of theft and corruption. All likewise blamed supervisors for failing to implement disciplinarymeasures. The result was demoralisation and cynicism among honest and hard-working staff. A nursing auxiliary expressed his moral outrage vividly:

> There are no disciplinary measures from top to bottom. Who is to discipline whom, when? Someone comes on duty drunk but he will never be disciplined. Are we not supposed to be disciplined? Where is this discipline? A known habitual loafer is never disciplined. Someone steals a patient's clothes. They know exactly who is responsible, but there will be no disciplinary action. They call a meeting of everyone and give a lecture on how to conduct ourselves.

A group of professional nurses also complained bitterly:

> There is a disease in management of not acting. Management knows the rotten potatoes andleaves them alone. If you report, you are regarded as a culprit. Then we all keep mum. Youcannot trust anyone.

The worst disciplinary problems are found among the cleaners, as one of them confirmed:

> Now we have corruption. Some do not work, others do. People are ungovernable. They just disappear; there is no discipline. They sign in for work and then go out, and at 3 p.m. theycome back just to sign out. Their supervisors know and do nothing. Some of them do their washing and ironing on the premises – even supervisors to this. Some of them are taxi owners and go to drive their taxis; others sell cassettes on the bridge.

Certain terms that have entered into the common

discourse at the hospital reflect the pervasive culture of flouting discipline and of supervisory apathy. Workers who cannot be found at their workstations are said to have gone 'over the bridge' – a reference to a bridge at the entrance to the hospital on top of which some 'loafers' join the throngs of hawkers selling a variety of goods, and over which others cross to reach the shebeens. Uyaziwa – He is known – refers to the attitude supervisors adopt in the face of habitual offenders; they are known to be lazy or drinkers, so there is no point in disciplining them. A 'banana' is a bribe, something that clerks in particular are reputed to be guilty of demanding from patients. Many workers complained that they were known as 'donkeys' who work hard, and that supervisors would pair a lazy worker with a donkey in order to ensure that the job is done.

One reason for the disciplinary paralysis at the hospital is the bureaucratic disciplinaryprocedures which have to be ratified by the provincial department of health. This example of the excessive centralisation of control results in endless delays and disciplinary failures. This undermines managerial authority, and many supervisors prefer to take the easy route and simply avoid trying to exert discipline (Tapson and Baker 2002: 4, 9-11)

More important, however, is the collapse of the old apartheid disciplinary regime in the face of worker resistance and democratic expectations, and a failure on the part of the institution to establish a new disciplinary regime. Virtually all interviewees referred to the NEHAWU strike in 1992 as a turning point. The strike began in June of that year whengeneral assistants at Baragwanath staged a wildcat walkout. It spread rapidly to otherhospitals, with some 8 000 workers on strike. The strike centred on wage demands and the absence of collective bargaining rights for public service workers. It dragged on for four months in the face of a hostile and intransigent old-order management, and was characterisedby escalating levels of worker violence. Twelve people were killed during the strike, with intimidation, assaults and arson directed against strikers and strike breakers alike, particularlyblack nurses who continued working. The union mobilised daily pickets and demonstrationsoutside Baragwanath, while management employed large numbers of scabs (Fenichel 1992: 11-3). When the strike was settled and the strikers returned to work at Baragwanath, they found they had to work side-by-side with the scabs whose services management refused to terminate. Both strikers and scabs had armed themselves in response to the violence of the conflict, and several of them continued to carry firearms at work. Supervisors were often afraid to discipline workers. The institution was left with a legacy of deep tension between workers. The strike had destroyed the harsh and anti-union disciplinary regime characteristic of the apartheid workplace in the public service, but nothing was established to take its place. A cleaner described the change:

> The hospital has been a mess since 1992. Workers used to fear their supervisors and run to dotheir work. When we came back after the 1992 strike we found cleaners and ward attendantswithout discipline, without training. We found trolleys everywhere. The ones who wereemployed as strike breakers are the problem – there is tension between them and other workers, and they are uncontrollable. They bring guns and alcohol to work. Now discipline is applied in a discriminatory way.

Speaking with indignation from within their status-conscious and authoritarian nursing culture, the CPNs associated this situation with the broader changes brought about by democratisation:

> When the ANC took over, everything became relaxed; you could do anything in the newdispensation .... The lowest categories control the hospital. Since the unions were introducedthe shop stewards have been running the hospital, but they cannot even write their names! They get out of hand and it is difficult to handle. Management is scared to discipline and control. The shop stewards confront and victimise the nurses. We also belong to a union but we do our job. Everyone barks at us. We have no dignity; we are degraded. There is supposedto be democracy, but not in the manner of Baragwanath.

The 1992 strike occurred at a watershed moment in the shift from the apartheid industrial relations order to a new democratic industrial relations order in the public service. Soon afterwards, trade unions were recognised, collective bargaining for the public service took place in the newly established Public Service Bargaining Council, and formal disciplinary and grievance procedures, including the right to trade union representation, were put in place. These changes have not facilitated the resolution of workers' problems, and a further unravelling of workplace order was manifested in an explosive and controversial countrywide series of wildcat strikes by nurses in 1995. While their immediate demand was for a fair payincrease, nurses also voiced grievances over shifts, grading, lack of workplace consultation and poor working conditions. They expressed an across-the-board hostility to all official worker organisations for failing to represent them adequately (Forrest 1996a, 1996b; see also Gwagwa and Webber 1995; Mantashe 1995; NEHAWU 1996).

By the time of our research, the trade unions at Chris Hani Baragwanath were meeting regularly with management to consult on issues of mutual concern. Each trade union had offices, and the majority trade union, NEHAWU, had three full-time shop stewards. However, despite the institutionalisation of trade unionism and workers' procedural rights in the institution, no proactive strategy has been established to build a new workplace regime, based on a new consensus about roles, rights and responsibilities. Thus discipline has been highly contested, with a minority of workers flouting any disciplinary control and backing this upwith threats of violence, supervisors abdicating disciplinary responsibility, and the majority of workers highly frustrated and resentful. In this fragmented and conflictual terrain, the trade unions themselves, particularly NEHAWU with its more militant traditions and base among the support workers, findthemselves locked into a negative role, using bureaucratic procedures to defend wrongdoers. A group of NEHAWU members expressed this concern forcefully:

> The union is defending those who are wrong. It must educate its members and shop stewards.
>
> There should be clear rules. What is the point of having lots of members while they are rotten?We are the real NEHAWU members. More are rotten, and they dominate. They like NEHAWU because when it says, "No, that is final". NEHAWU delivers, but some people take advantage.

As the nurses observe, the broader transition from apartheid to a democratic order has plunged the workplace regime into crisis. A similar process of decomposition occurred in the manufacturing sector during and after the transition, but there market pressures tended to impel managers to adopt proactive strategies for establishing a new workplace order (Von Holdt 2003b: 238-40). At Chris Hani Baragwanath Hospital, in contrast, market pressures do not play a role, and neither management nor the Department of Health have the capacity or the expertise to develop a more strategic response. Indeed, the institution has what is essentially a personnel administration department which was designed for the apartheid-era workplace instead of a genuine human resources department with the strategic capacity to envisage and work towards a new workplace order. This does not seem to disturb ANC politicians such as the Minister of Finance who routinely continue to denounce the behaviour and ethics of public service workers rather then grapple with the structural causes ofworkplace disorder (Von Holdt 2003a).

Work Organisation and Skills Formation

The silo structures of management, reinforced by a general lack of managerial capacity,create a fragmented work organisation which generates tremendous inefficiencies and frustration at the site of actual health care delivery – the wards. While the most senior CPN isin charge of the ward, she has no authority over ward clerks, cleaners and ward attendants. This leads to frequent conflict over who is supposed to do what and who has the authority to issue instructions. A nursing supervisor explained that the demarcation between different categories of worker creates 'grey areas' which have to be negotiated. For example, if blood is required the doctor may have to fetch it himself if a ward attendant or nursing auxiliary refuses, because it is not strictly part of their job description. The CPNs described the difficulties of trying 'to work with those who are managed fromfar away'. Non-nursing staff such as cleaners, ward clerks and ward attendants responded to their requests 'with the refrain that "I do not fall under a nurse"'.

Ward clerks experienced their separation from the nursing function as a form of isolation. One said, 'We are isolated from daily ward life, and only do the boring repetitive paperwork for the wards'. Like other categories of staff, they described tensions over supervision, claiming that nursing supervisors provoked and interfered with them 'by always talking in a sarcastic way to us'. Virtually all levels of staff complained about a lack of respect between categories. As one CPN acknowledged, 'We call the ward attendants uneducated, whereas we know the reasons why someone lacks the education; it is no fault of their own'.

As far as the ward attendants, ward clerks and nursing auxiliaries were concerned, their reluctance to co-operate was a response to the excessive workload, their frustration that their skills were not recognised, and the lack of opportunities for training and advancement. Theyall expressed keenness to expand their jobs by taking on more skilled tasks. This might openup prospects for training and advancement and end their current frustration. As a ward clerk explained, 'I find my routine work very boring and demotivating. I have been in my post for ten years. I need change. There is no career path for us'. Yet the hospital was pursuing the opposite strategy, cutting down on its training. For example, the training of nursing auxiliaries had stopped, and the hospital was recruiting fromthe ranks of those who had already paid for their own training externally. Likewise, thenursing college attached to Chris Hani Baragwanath was training professional nurses bytaking 'new students from the location, but they do not take us, they do not appreciate our contribution'. As with the ward attendants, the nursing auxiliaries were required to orient auxiliaries who came from outside as well as train the student nurses, 'but tomorrow she is my senior, telling me what to do'. This problem was aggravated by the fact that staff shortages made it impossible to release staff for training.

These inefficiencies, frustrations and conflicts experienced in the wards were replicated atthe broader level, in the relationship between the wards and other departments and activities in the institution. Thus nurses complained about shortages of vital equipment. Equipment that was sent away for repair, or orders for new equipment, would disappear with no explanation about what was happening. Linen shortages were a perennial problem. The pharmacy was inefficient so nurses had to repeat their trips to it. The IT system was a shambles so ward clerks spent much of their time as messengers, taking forms from one point to another. All of these problems made the workers in the wards feel that there was a managerial vacuum.

Impact on Morale and Work Culture

The overwhelming impression, from the CEO who explained that he was unable to get the hospital clean to the cleaners who complained that they were never consulted, was a sense of disempowerment, a sense that nothing could change. A nursing auxiliary spoke with deepbitterness about his sense of alienation from his calling:

> I have served with every energy I have got. I feel neglected. When I wake up in the morning my soul is not up-to-date; I feel sick and I do not want to come to work. We do the dirtiest jobs of all. That is fine, that is our training. But the worst is the salary. The last resort is to resignfrom hospital and sell vegetables in the township.

Frustration about the declining quality of health care delivery at Chris Hani Baragwanath, and their own inability to perform their jobs well, was felt to be profoundly undermining. As one nurse explained, 'We used to be proud to work at Bara; even the way you walked to work showed your pride. Now you are just ashamed'.

The Union Project for Reconstruction

It was in this context of extreme frustration and demoralisation that NALEDI worked together with the trade unions and staff in the Surgical Department to develop a set of proposals to transform the way in which work was organised. Given that the over-riding problem articulated by staff was the managerial vacuum that they experienced, and that without an effective management structure there was no prospect of implementing anychanges, the proposals devoted considerable attention to developing more effective management structures and practices. The underlying assumption was that more effective management and work organisation would enable better use to be made of existing resources and staff; staff shortages could be accurately assessed and strategies developed to address them. The key elements in the Business Plan (2003) were:

— The silo structures of management were to be replaced with an integrated andaccountable managerial structure. A general manager for the Surgical Department would be responsible for the effective functioning of the entire department. A ward manager for each ward would be responsible for managing all operations within the ward.

— Human resources management should be brought out of the administration block and intothe workplace by establishing a new position of human resources officer for the Surgical Department, whose role would be to manage the implementation of many of theprocesses described below.

— The fragmented work organisation in the wards would be replaced with an integrated work organisation. This would be based on a team-working approach where working relationships and joint problem-solving processes would be established, and then assessing staff shortages.

— A joint management-labour process would be implemented, to establish a new disciplinary regime with mutually understood roles and codes of conduct to which supervisors, shop stewards and staff would be held accountable.

— New business systems would be implemented so that cost centre and quality auditaccountabilities could be put in place.

— Once the new system of ward management and integrated work organisation was functioning properly, more advanced work organisation would be developed and implemented. It would be based on the recognition of skills and multi-skilling of the wardattendants, nursing auxiliaries and ward clerks, whose numbers would ultimately be increased so as to relieve the pressures on the professional nurses. Training and careerpathing would be developed.

These proposals were adopted by the management of the hospital and accepted by the provincial Department of Health at the beginning of 2003. One of the hospital superintendents was appointed to fill the surgical general manager position (without reducing any of his other responsibilities!). The new management team consisting of the superintendent, the chief clinician, the nursing assistant director and the nursing and clericalcorridor supervisors started meeting regularly to put in place the conditions for implementingthe proposals. It took the entire year to draw up the job descriptions for the new positions, win departmental approval, advertise, interview and fill them – a measure of how cumbersomeand under-resourced these procedures are. Nonetheless, in the context of the general institutional paralysis and disempowerment, this progress is counted by all involved as a genuine success for the project. In the course of the year, the management team also began tograpple with operational issues, providing a forum for beginning to empower managers and holding them accountable. The key drivers of the project have been NEHAWU, NALEDI, and specific individuals in the surgical management team. While all the trade unions at Chris

Hani Baragwanath Hospital have played a significant role in developing the proposals and providing the project with credibility, NEHAWU has played a particularly important role in putting political pressure on the Gauteng Department of Health to take the project seriously, using meetings with the Premier, the MEC for Health, and departmental managers to good effect. This has been critically important, since while health officials have given full verbal support, in practice – particularly in relation to securing financial support – their support has been somewhatambiguous.

NALEDI has played a central role in conceptualising and winning support for the project among staff and managers, as well as at provincial level. Indeed, the lack of managerial capacity in the institution has led NALEDI to provide ongoing support and advice not only tolabour but also to management. NALEDI advisers, for example, attend the SurgicalDepartment managerial team meetings as full participants. At the same time, individualmanagers in the managerial team have been key change agents in their contribution to shapingthe proposals, their commitment to implementation, and their role in persuading the institutional management to adopt and support them.

The modest progress so far has therefore depended on the leadership provided by keymanagers and trade unionists, as well as on the capacity for innovation which NALEDI represents within the trade union movement. Future progress will depend on the continued support of these actors. In the view of NALEDI, when it comes to the concrete implementation of change in the work process, the indignation and frustration of the health care workers – which is an index of their commitment to good quality health care – will be avitally important driving force for new ways of working. The apartheid workplace regime at Chris Hani Baragwanath Hospital was both similar to and different from the workplace regime in private-sector industry. It was characterised byracial domination, the absence of worker and trade union rights, and managerial despotism. However, it was a more bureaucratic, administrative and rules-based system of management. The composition of the workforce was more complex and differentiated along racial and skills lines, which created particular challenges and tensions for black trade unionism. Most distinctive was the fact that the biggest contingent of professional workers, the nursing staff, was almost entirely black. The hospital was completely dependent on their labour, yet their ideology of professionalism and self-improvement, and tight control by SANA, made themless susceptible to trade union organisation or militant action. During the 1992 strike, for example, they continued working in the face of militant pressure and intimidation fromstriking support staff. It was only in 1995 that nurses themselves went on strike in utter desperation at their working conditions. A final distinguishing feature was that widespread trade unionism and the winning of trade union rights came a decade later than in the privatesector, making them phenomena of the transition rather than of the struggle against apartheid.

With the transition came the rapid growth of public service trade unionism, frequent consultation with government and highly centralised collective bargaining. As a result of this and other factors, there was a weak tradition of workplace organisation and engagement with management, in contrast to the long-established private-sector trade unions. Further contrastsare also noticeable at Chris Hani Baragwanath Hospital – the workforce composition makes for more pluralistic and fragmented trade unionism, which reproduces professional tensions (for example, between nurses and cleaners); at the same time there is a less antagonistic relationship between trade unions and management, as they are united by an ideology of public service, however fractious their relations may be.

The triple dimensions of the South African transition (Von Holdt 2003b) have therefore had a contradictory impact on the Chris Hani Baragwanath workplace. Democratic rights have been firmly established: workers have trade union rights and access to disciplinary and grievance procedures, the minimum wage has increased, and the wage gap between bottomand top has diminished dramatically – from 62:1 in 1989 to 16:1 in 1998 (Adler 1998). On the other hand, the racist, bureaucratic, hierarchical and authoritarian management of the apartheid era has changed much less. Much of the racial tension and despotism of the old order may have been eroded, and the racial structure of management has shifted moresubstantially than in the private sector. However, most staff are still administered as disempowered objects, as they were under apartheid, rather than as human agents who haveemotional lives and ideas about work, and the capacity to negotiate and consult with managers. The apartheid legacy is also felt in the financial differentiation between previouslyblack and previously white hospitals. The result is poor working conditions and poor service for the generally poorer residents of black townships next to which the previously black hospitals are located, compared to the racially mixed urban and suburban population served by the previously white hospitals.

The economic transition has reinforced these results. While the public service workplace is relatively insulated from market pressures, the budgetary constraints that accompany a rigid commitment to macro-economic 'stability' have, when combined with the restructuring of the health budget, placed the institutional fabric under enormous pressure. Workers now labour under an impossible workload

– far greater than private sector workers who labour under market pressures – which severely compromises both their own health and the quality of health-care delivery to the working-class communities they serve.

The combined impact of apartheid remnants and the reduction of budgets has produced a decomposition of the workplace regime, characterised by a profound disorder and paralysis,which management lacks any kind of strategy or capacity to address. There is much evidence that this situation is not unique, but is widespread in public hospitals, particularly those formerly classified as black (IMMSA 1995; Commission of Inquiry 1999; Landman, Mouton and Nevhutalu 2001; Baker and Tapson 2003).

This situation raises broader questions about the legacy of apartheid in the health sector. Chris Hani Baragwanath Hospital in particular, and the public hospitals more generally, are overwhelmingly the providers of health services to those who are not covered by private medical aid – that is, to the poor and mostly black majority of our society. Even if the restructuring of the health budget improves the delivery of health clinics and district hospitals as is intended, this is unlikely to reduce the pressure of patient numbers on the tertiaryhospitals (Department of Health 2003a: 5-6). Indeed, there are strong arguments to be madethat improving primary health care results in increased rather than reduced referrals to thespecialist health care provided by such institutions. Yet current government policy is leadingto the destruction of their institutional capacity, and starving them of the managerial resourcesthey need in order to respond innovatively. The apartheid bifurcation of health service provision into different levels of care for white and black is being replicated in the new South Africa, not only in the form of lower levels of funding for previously black hospitals but also in the form of radically different levels of care for those who can afford private medical aid and those who cannot. At Chris Hani Baragwanath Hospital, the only sign of an innovative response to this crisis is the transformation project initiated by the trade unions. As this book was going to publication, the Gauteng MEC for Health mandated NALEDI to facilitate a strategic planningprocess for the institution as a whole – hopefully a sign that the broader crisis of hospital.

5

Case Study: Aspects of Hospital Administration in UK

CONTROL MECHANISMS AND STRATEGIES IN U.K. HOSPITALS

To control' is the last of Fayol's five elements of management, the others being to forecast and plan, to organise and build, to command and to coordinate or bind together all corporate activity. Henri Fayol was a comtemporary of Taylor although details of his pioneering work on management theory were published only in French and only one year before Taylor's death. Obviously his major paper, 'Administration Industrielle et Generate (1916), appeared too late to influence Taylor's theories.

Control has always been of central concern in all organisations from the Armed Forces to the Christian Church and from commercial business to professional bodies. It is the mechanism for ensuring that objectives are met and necessary corrections and adjustments in performance occur to make that happen. The concept of control, say Porter et al., involves the notion of regulation and requires four basic elements, namely:

— standards or objectives
— monitoring systems

— comparison devices
— action devices to correct deviant performance

Put simply, controlling is the process by which management sees if what did happen was what was supposed to happen and the making of necessary adjustments. However, we believe that the notion of negative feedback tends to underemphasize the concept of forward control and 'proactivity', whereby the organisation endeavours to prescribe future events by means of specific intervention strategies linked to the planning process. Through the study of past outcomes of planning, recurrent mistakes may be avoided and the occurrence of deviation avoided by anticipation. For example, during a surgical operation, the anaesthetist will take corrective action through monitoring feedback information, to balance the administration of anaesthesia and other drugs to maintain the required level of unconsciousness and various body functions. His or her strategy, however, will have been planned in advance and based upon the experience of outcomes of many different patients undergoing similar operations. The plan will aim to prevent wide deviations occurring in the parameters monitored and the subsequent need for unplanned action.

At the same time the technique employed by the surgeon will seek to minimize postoperative pain and discomfort, help prevent complications during recovery and so ease and hasten the return to normality. This is a further example of proactivity and planning in the process of control. Compared with surgery, control mechanisms in organisations appear far more complex and less predictable since in this case we are not seeking to control physical functions of employees but their behaviour. Indeed it could be argued, say Cooper and Makin, that behaviour is what the employee sells to the organisation. If we accept this, it follows that organisations take different employees, holding disparate views on matters not directly related to their work and expect them, in spite of that, to comply with prescribed patterns of working practice and with organisational rules and norms of behaviour in response to a variety of control mechanisms. Organisations have been classified by Etzioni into three ideal types, depending on the particular control mechanisms used, namely:

Coercive: where force can be legitimately used such as prisons, armies and others.

Utilitarian: the basis of control here is remuneration and in its most blatant form is manifested in piece work, work contracts on a daily basis, use of time cards, low basic pay with the requirement to work overtime to achieve reasonable take-home pay. More sophisticated examples would include a low interest mortgage tied to job holding, or a tied cottage, which in turn is linked with 'satisfactory' performance. *Normative or moral controls:* applicable to religions, political or voluntary organisations and to a certain degree such controls may be applied in professional organisations where normative behaviour is identified with professional image. In practice, the influence of all three types tends to coalesce in a cultural norm for each organisation or each occupational group or department. Frequently in large organisations different norms apply in different sections of the same organisation. For example, the use of time or clock cards is both coercive and utilitarian in that latecoming is usually 'punished' by the deduction of one quarter of an hour's pay for every interval of lateness of up to three minutes. Thus, for a worker who 'clocks-on', to be unaccountably more than nine minutes late means that at least one hour's pay is deducted as well as being faced with the prospect of disciplinary proceedings. Moreover, a worker cannot make up the hour at the end of the day by voluntarily working longer as a 'flexitime' worker would be able to do.

For this he or she would require authorized overtime, paid at the agreed rate, and that would be worked to suit the needs of management, not of the worker!

Whereas a salaried worker arriving late may well be able to make up the lost time by local arrangement or convention, the moral (normative) pressure brought to bear by the anticipation of the manager's expression of disapproval or more particularly of peer group pressure to conform to group behavioural norms may exert a powerful controlling influence on latecoming. In this example the personal views of the individual employee with regard to time-keeping are of no concern to the organisation but behaviour is; the organisation is rightly concerned that each employee arrives at work at an agreed time. Other important aspects of behaviour can be viewed in this way, such as the requirements to demonstrate a duty of care to the employer, to work to the best of one's ability or to refrain from racial, sexual or religious prejudice at work. Organisational control then is aimed at maintaining acceptable behaviour at work and not at changing workers' personalities.

Indeed we hold the view that a worker's personality is a wholly owned set of entities and characteristics and is rightly regarded by employers as inviolable. The link between personality (input) and behaviour (output) is personal belief. It is an abiding human experience that belief is a state of mind; a conviction of the truth of some state of affairs whether supported by objective evidence or not. 'Now faith is the substance of things hoped for, the evidence of things not seen.' Belief can produce stubbornness or flexibility, the rejection of a pay increase or its acceptance. It can reject the most moderate control proposals or it can accept them, even suggest them, depending on what it perceives to be reality. The beliefs of employees then will need to be addressed by the organisation in so far as beliefs directly influence behaviour where such behaviour seriously threatens the reasonable operation of the employment contract. Ultimately, an employee who is unhappy with the aims or methods of his or her organisation may have to consider the option of changing employment should personal value systems be compromized by required behaviour at work. Animal research is one such example of what we have in mind. It is likely that some of the causes of the dysfunctions of organisational control structures arise not only through employees' personal constructs which relate more to individuals than to groups, but through the shared belief that in fealty to certain powerful, key individuals who do not recognize the controls or who cannot be bound by them, lies the safest way for the development or survival of their hitherto occupational autonomy. One particular strategy is to conform excessively to control procedures to the exclusion of overall organisational objectives—so-called bureaucratic behaviour, working to rule, or goal displacement.Further types identified by Porter include the use of invalid data both with regard to what has been achieved and what may be achieved.

Inflation of workload returns is an example of the former while resistance to proposed manning levels or budgetary provisions illustrate the latter. Since NHS managers are now providing much more information for management information systems it follows that dysfunctions in control systems at data source will have far-reaching consequences throughout the organisations, in planning, staffing, budgeting and ultimately in performance. Resistance to control systems may arise because imposed control necessarily limits individual freedom for the employee to take the intrinsic rewards associated with work and which are perceived to be part of the psychological contract of employment. On the other hand, acceptance of control may occur because perceived needs are met or value systems upheld by the particular controls used. Workers may agree about the need for and legitimacy of the control system, for example that pilfering should be stopped, that poor workers and bad work should not be ignored and that there is a system for recognizing good work and the contribution of ideas and extra effort to the organisation. Factors identified by Lawler regarding success in control systems may be related to Porter's four basic elements of control referred to earlier. For example, while standards that are set too low tend to be disregarded as irrelevant, the highest possible standards of achievement may be perceived as unattainable. Both types may be expected to engender resistance. Moderately high standards on the other hand are seen to be most effective in motivation particularly if the individuals to whom they apply have had opportunity to contribute in setting them. Unilateral standard setting by management may be regarded as coercion, whereas motivation, in its most effective sense, arises out of a person's internalized desire to achieve and may be regarded as stemming from the individual belief system which has adopted a personal norm by which to guide behaviour.

Success is thus linked to the individual's sense of involvement and will have a particular bearing on whether the 'spirit' rather than the 'letter' of the standard is attained. The manner of performance monitoring may also be contentious. If employees believe that such monitoring does not fairly reflect work effort or that it is subjective, their willingness to accept it will be correspondingly reduced. Again the comparison of actual with expected performance would appear best left to the employee as this seems to be the strongest motivation in maintaining performance. In many industrial operations, as part of a programme of job enrichment, self-control in the form of quality control checking has been made the employees' responsibility with resulting improvements in productivity and of the 'them and us' mentality that had previously existed on both sides. Of course if the employee himself is placed in the feedback loop it is he who must make the necessary corrections to the system.

If he is a manager it becomes his decision to, say, leave a post unfilled in order to reach a budgetary target, his decision to buy in bulk to obtain a discount, his decision to rearrange staff deployment in order to meet new demand without additional resources. It is also his responsibility to make and support a case for additional resources where these are necessary. Where true, straight-line accountability exists in an organisation such delegation is not only possible, it is desirable and, moreover, its absence is indicative of dysfunction. However, the managerial task is to exercise sufficient depth and breadth of control so that short-term performance is always seen as contributing to long-term objectives. Both may be valid, but long-term plans may call for tactical changes, redefinition of standards and the recognition that each organisational control system is probably vested inside another whose span of control and breadth of perspective is greater than that of its subordinates. Clearly there is no universal model of organisational control.

Differences in function, in technology and in staffing make this inevitable. Moreover, it would appear evident that organisation structures, like culture, evolve to meet specific task objectives and that, since control mechanisms form part of the organisation's character, they are best determined also within the organisation, rather than prescribed from outside. It is also necessary that they are congruent with long-term objectives rather than short-term expediency and permit appropriate autonomy and growth for those people who work in the organisation and for whom such rewards are desirable. Having examined briefly something of the theoretical concepts of organisation control we now turn to consider ways in which control is implemented in organisations and, in particular, the NHS and to suggest ways in which such control may be improved. As we have seen, control is integral to the management process and it is therefore sensible to devise an organisational structure that reflects this concept. By this we mean that all officers that are able to exercise control are accounted for in the organisation chart. The traditional hierarchical chart appears to us to have two weaknesses. First, it universally fails to convey the cultural dynamics of an organisation, tending always to impose a bureaucratic rigidity on staff structure whether this is appropriate or not. Second, because of the importance of role holding in bureaucracies such charts tend to emphasize the boxes (roles) rather than the adjoining lines (relationships).

However, some workers, almost exclusively medical staff, believe their clinical function to be properly outside and separate from their organisational one. They decline to accept that they can be totally accountable to a general manager, whether medically qualified or not. Further difficulties arise where some of these medical workers are themselves managers of other occupational or professional groups who would otherwise be amenable to the principles of general management but who feel obliged to support, or who are coerced into supporting, a covert guerrilla war aimed at preventing the loss of hitherto unchallenged professional dominance. It appears to us that an important plank of the Griffiths proposals was that doctors, who commit resources in the NHS, accept managerial accountability for the totality of their actions rather than just take part in certain management functions such as planning team membership or deciding on the purchase of medical equipment. Clinical freedom is, after all, bounded by the rationality of corporate planning including the planned financial consequences of clinical decisions. Without a commitment to work within the concept of accountability clinical budgeting and even effective planning will become impossible. Absolute clinical freedom, however, is a myth. Nickson suggests that each person should have only one line manager. Others may have functional authority to give instructions or guidance concerning particular areas of work but staff should remain ultimately accountable to a single line boss. In managerial terms the professional designation of manager and subordinate may well be different and interchangeable in different areas of the organisation. In other words they are not required to be members of the same profession or occupational group although in many instances it is sensible that they should be. However, when management appointments are truly based on management qualifications and ability many of the problems associated with the relationships between different professional groups will begin to disappear. 'In the NHS', says Nickson, 'where so much is done by teams of different specialists, and when the decisions of one person can affect directly the resources of another, accountable management will require a major rethinking of organisational relationships.' We believe that this should involve determining not only 'to whom' but 'for what' one is accountable.

Often, job descriptions which are expected to contain such information are compiled in rather passive terms and consist merely of lists of activities in which the post holder is to engage. It would be useful if, as far as possible, all statements were couched in terms of their desired outcomes and referred to quantifiable output requirements from post holders. Although in these circumstances job descriptions would require regular updating they would provide a reason for each role relationship by stating what those relationships were meant to achieve. In this way the job description would more appropriately describe the basic framework of organisational control.

Authority

Accountability may be defined as 'the obligation to act', whereas authority, which must always accompany it, is seen as 'the power or right to act' and must be commensurate with the level of responsibility given. Although some writers attribute different meanings to the terms 'accountability' and 'responsibility', such differentiation seems to us to be of academic interest only. The choice of term may be left to organisational preference; both imply binding obligation. At present the term 'accountability' is favoured in the NHS, no doubt due to the necessary attempt to change organisational mores. In an organisational context we take both terms to be interchangeable. While accountability is an obligation placed on an individual as a post holder, authority is power given to the role itself rather than to the person. The authority vested in a managerial position', say Koontz and O'Donnell, 'is the right to use discretion, the right to create and maintain an environment for the performance of individuals working together in groups.' The true implication of this ability to create is then not autocratic.' It is, they assert, 'no accident that "authority" derives from the same Latin root that "author" does.' There are two commonly held misconceptions with regard to authority and accountability.

The first is that authority is absolute and that if only the NHS had 'strong' management its organisational problems could be solved at a stroke. Of the many authors we have studied none holds to this view regarding organisational control. Such problems seem to exist in all organisations the world over including those behind the Iron Curtain. Not only does absolute power corrupt, but the application of absolute power does not work either, whether we consider the policies of Hitler, the Americans in Vietnam, the Pol Pot regime in Kampuchea or the Shah of Iran. Authority is ultimately based upon recognition and acceptance by those under it. Moreover, this is not a once-and-for-all endorsement but a continuing process based on the acceptance of policy and its interpretation—hence the particular difficulty with organisational change. As with politics, management may be regarded as the 'art of the possible' subsumed as it is, with an organisational and legal framework and with agreed goals and objectives. Organisational control, as an integral part of the management process, is no less constrained.

Delegation

The second misconception that may frequently arise is that responsibility (or accountability) may be delegated. This is emphatically not so. Such an obligation may only be transferred by changing the employment contract such as occurs at a change of post—a promotion or demotion. Delegation, on the other hand, may be defined as 'the act of empowering to act for another' but in organisational terms there is a broad spectrum of meaning in this word. At one end of the spectrum are considerations of structure which may be enshrined in role definitions and job descriptions. At the other end lies the discretion of managerial techniques of style and of practice.

From this definition comes the notion that what is actually delegated is the authority to act for another, not the responsibility for the outcome of that action. Indeed, Hicks argues that the delegation of authority to act may well increase a manager's responsibility, since in addition he then carries a consequently heavier commitment to supervise his delegate. However, this view appears confused, reflecting a muddled distinction between supervision and delegation. We prefer to link delegation with decision-making. 'Authority is delegated when enterprise discretion is vested in a subordinate by a supervisor.' There is a limit to the number of persons a manager can effectively supervise and for whom he can make decisions. Once this limit is passed, authority must be delegated to subordinates who will make decisions within the area of their assigned duties. Indeed, without delegation of authority, formal organisations could not exist. Therefore, the process of delegating authority is a constant feature of formal organisation. However, not only is delegation a formal strategy of control, it is also something that may be subject to dysfunction and can weaken overall control. In mechanistic systems similar to the rational bureaucratic model of Weber, the problems and tasks which face the concern as a whole are typically broken down into specialities. This is certainly a characteristic of the NHS.

Each individual (or group) carries out his assigned tasks as something apart from the overall purpose of the organisation as a whole. Moreover, the mechanistic model tends to define technical methods, duties and powers precisely and places a high value on precision and demarcation. Interactions within the working organisations follow vertical lines, i.e. between superiors and subordinates. This hierarchy of command is maintained by the assumption that the only person who knows or should know all about the organisation is the person at the top. If this seems oversimplified in today's world, one has only to examine the tendency in the NHS for certain organisational members, particularly professionals who are not bureaucratic office-holders, to by-pass normal channels and to seek to appeal directly to the top, hoping that delegated policy-making or decisions will be over-ruled or changed. At times of rapid change or where there is a perceived requirement for more control by the top hierarchy, an increased delegation of authority may be instituted. Selznick argues that delegation leads to increased training in specialized competences, improves the employee's capability and narrows the gap between organisational goals and actual achievement. This then leads to more delegation. However, delegation increases departmentalisation and this leads in time to a divergence of interests among the sub-units in the organisation. Sub-unit goals grow in precedence and their members tend to become dependent more upon the survival and prestige of the sub-unit than of the organisation. More training courses are organised. Sub-units compete for resources and otherwise conflict. Organisational decisions become constrained by considerations of internal strategy particularly if there is little internalisation of organisational goals by participants. As the difference now grows between goals and achievement more delegation is called for to solve the problem. For example, the bringing in of someone to deal with the problem, an intermediary, a communications specialist or a liaison officer. Child believes many writers have seen the main contribution of organisation structure to be in the means it provides for controlling behaviour.

In fact the conventional organisation chart expressed the official channels of control. He sees control as essentially concerned with regulating the activities within one organisation so that they are in accord with expectations established in policies, plans and targets and argues that the achievement of control has always been a managerial priority. Departmental heads have taken the demonstration of their 'authority' over their employees as a basic criterion of their competence to manage rather than say, goal attainment, high productivity or successful coordination with other managers. Of Fayol's five basic managerial functions, Child believes more has been written on control than on any other, yet the literature on delegation is relatively small.This is because in the past many managers have been inclined to equate control with close direction and delegated with reluctance, feeling secure only where subordinates' discretion had been effectively limited by a combination of job descriptions, budgetary controls, costing systems, work study, manuals of procedure, standard operating systems, exception reporting systems and similar devices. The resulting low motivation this produces in highly trained and expectant staff may give rise to the notion of coordination as a managerial concept (and problem). This was certainly a prominent feature of the 1974 NHS reorganisation. Coordination is easily seen as a supervisory rather than a managerial function and these problems associated with delegation again illustrate the trust-control dilemma discussed by Handy and to which we have already referred. That is, close prescription and supervision on the one hand (but with low self-motivation) is balanced against the costs and benefits of self-regulation by workers and relative freedom on the other (with the possible loss of control by management). How can this dilemma be resolved?

There are a number of techniques and strategies which organisations may adopt depending on particular circumstances and the nature of the tasks in hand. We discuss below three techniques which concentrate on the process of the organisation and which may be helpful in setting defined limits within which control and decision-making may be adequately delegated. These are the processes of work study, operation research and budgetary control. We then consider three strategies which may be regarded as facilitative approaches to delegation, to control and to staff management, namely management by objectives (MBO), performance appraisal and performance related pay. Finally we discuss briefly the need for adequate personnel policies to provide a framework for good management practice.

Work Study

The scientific study of work, usually known as organisation and methods study or O and M, is another surviving legacy from F.W. Taylor's theories of Scientific Management. As we have already discussed, his views stemmed from his belief that both workers and their managers were ignorant with respect to the organisation of work and need the intervention of a trained engineer who would, after observation and measurement, scientifically calculate and prescribe the most efficient method to be used in each working situation. Fortunately, there are several differences between Taylor's early approach and the practice of O and M today. Firstly, in 1954 the Management Services Division of Her Majesty's Treasury could say:

> The result of O and M work is advice. The manager or administrator remains responsible for the efficient execution of the work in his/her charge. Any attempt to give O and M proposals the force of instruction would set up undesirable conflicts of authority'.

The second difference is that where Taylor was concerned to establish the maximum workload, short of fatigue, that a worker could tolerate in a day (and therefore the highest take-home pay) our current approach considers the optimum workload; not what a person can achieve but what he should achieve given all the relevant facts surrounding him and his work. Thirdly, Taylor's preoccupation with profit maximisation has given way to a concern for cost minimisation. Other developments within management services departments have included a general move away from piece-rated pay, a greater emphasis on quality control and the setting of quality standards and a concern for the purpose or reason for any organisation's existence rather than a zeal for method study and for rated performance. O and M staff are generally members of a department of management services. As such they are frequently asked to examine and advise on a wide variety of organisational problems, many of which may be unsuitable for the traditional clipboard and stopwatch observations.

Bottom Up Investigations

The detailed analysis of the working in any department can involve several trained observers and will be very time-consuming and therefore expensive. Managers will be concerned that the potential improvements identified by the study will be feasible and broadly justify the study. The bottom up approach begins with the agreement of the terms of reference and discussion of methods to be adopted with the relevant management. The O and M team's first task is to learn as much about the department as possible, its structure, its work and how it fits into the organisation.

The discussion should include any criticisms of the department that have been made and any problems or constraints that have been identified by managers and staff. Local records will also be examined and in due course a proposed study outline is submitted for local approval. There are different approaches for different types of departments. The analysis of an outpatient clinic will be different from that of a hospital laundry. For example, it may be required that work be rated for the purpose of agreeing standard workrates in the laundry since the processing of work is highly deterministic given reliable equipment and a continuous supply of work. In this example it is usual for the precise detail of each separate procedure to be discussed with the operatives themselves to ascertain the easiest, most comfortable and most efficient way of doing each job. This has been called Method Study, the origins of which can be traced right back to Taylor. After agreeing working practice the next step is to define a standard work-rate. For example, how many items of laundry can be processed in one hour allowing for a number of identifiable factors.

No worker is able to sustain a maximum possible work rate for an entire day. It is common to fix the standard work-rate at a percentage of the average maximum which is calculated by a combination of observation and negotiation with the workers themselves. At all times the quality of output is an important factor in such calculations. There are many local factors that may affect work-rate such as machine speeds and reliability, manning levels, working conditions, experience of workers and the particular combination of duties each worker is required to perform each day. These all produce a need for adequate rest and relaxation to be taken into account in order that quality and quantity of output may be optimized. In some cases a bonus payment scheme will be built into the agreement and will apply to workers who exceed the agreed standard rate. However, in recent years some such schemes have been renegotiated due to a shortage of money and the need to remain competitive in the face of possible privatisation. In the outpatient department, office areas and paramedical departments there may still be a place for Method Study and the need for reorganisation of working practice. We believe that the success of suggestions or reports that may emerge from such O and M analysis will depend upon three factors. Who invites the O and M team in; who contributes most to the suggested improvements; who is seen to benefit from the changes that are finally recommended. If, for example, an O and M study is the result of a staff suggestion as part of a change management projectthen the outcome becomes useful information for the staff of the department since they continue to own their problems. If, on the other hand, management seeks to impose its reported findings, much goodwill and efficiency may be lost. Other strategies will need to be employed to convince workers of the need for change in order to prevent the perceptions of injustice from diverting energy into disruptive or non-productive behaviour.

Top Down Analysis

Although there are many other areas apart from the laundry where the bottom up approach may be used the top down approach has become popular because it is generally cheaper to do and may be easier to interpret when comparing report findings from different but inter-reacting departments. Top down studies concentrate on outputs and are concerned with departmental policy, workload, staffing and non-staffing costs. They generally make comparisons with other similar departments in much the same way as performance indicators attempt to permit us to do. Although this approach is faster and less expensive than the bottom up method, ultimate success is dependent upon the same factors. An adversarial stance by the O and M team will be provocative to departmental managers who are the ones who are required to produce data for analysis. Workers may feel a top down based report may lack credibility because they have seen no measurements or observations made of their work. O and M work at this level may become less relevant in future. Management has often used these approaches in order simply to learn what is actually going on in a department about which it may know practically nothing.

Management information systems will, in the future, fill this considerable gap, and help to increase the quality of the dialogue between tiers of management and therefore to increase and refine the levels and mechanisms of control.

Operational Research (OR)

'Operational Research is the science of planning and executing an operation to make the most economical use of the resources available.' It is characterized by a quantitative approach to management and covers a range of mathematical methods that are applicable to planning and running an enterprise. These include, for example, the application of probability theory to, say, the pricing of guaranteed goods for sales (a simple calculation) to the complex mathematical model-building and simulation using computers.

The aim of OR is always to choose the course which yields the best results for the whole organisation, to increase organisational effectiveness and to identify the external variables that are likely to exist in a variety of forms and which will influence the outcome of all operations. The optimisation of methods by operational research, therefore, inevitably constrains the freedom of managers in order that their operations become increasingly congruent with those of the organisation as a whole. Although the origins of OR can be traced back to the Industrial Revolution, it is recognized that most of the OR techniques and strategies were developed during and after the Second World War.

Initially, large-scale projects were selected for operational research because increased effectiveness would result not only in large-scale economies but in better control in areas where control was enormously difficult to achieve, e.g. the movement of large numbers of military personnel and items of equipment overseas. The development of computers after the war permitted OR to be applied more widely and to include mathematical modelling and dynamic simulation of working problems. These techniques are equally applicable to small local situations as well as to large global problems and to matters of operational significance as well as to the determination of policy. In practice they are more likely to help the manager directly rather than individual workers although of course, workers are ultimately affected by its outcome. OR, then, is a collection of management tools which is used to assist decision-making.

OR in Health Care

Some of the specific areas addressed by OR include the analysis of queueing—characteristically applicable in the NHS; stock control— relevant in all organisations; forecasting—the frequency of occurrence of future events; project management—using network analysis and transportation problems. All these areas are relevant to the Health Service at different levels. For example, the emphasis on stock control and purchasing is now centred at regional and national level. However, local (district) managers require predictable control parameters for ensuring a safe supply of stock. Regular transport runs may be optimized by the use of a simple form of linear programming. Before any formulae can be applied or computer assistance obtained, data concerning the task to be analysed has first to be collected. When studying a queueing problem for example, observation and measurement of the arrival rate of patients in, say an outpatient department, will have to be made. This work would be undertaken either by members of an OR department or by management services personnel using OR as an appropriate tool. It may well be that some useful observations by managers can be helpful. For example, by recording the work arrival pattern for each quarter of an hour throughout the day for several days any daily or weekly periodicity will be shown. The manager may then be able to respond more sensitively to workload demand by appropriate staff deployment. Although most managers might argue that they are aware of such matters, it is the quantitative discipline that OR brings which often reveals unsuspected facts as well as facilitating quantitative answers to problems, e.g. specified additional resources to meet quantified need!

In a more complex situation a department may be experiencing difficulties in completing its work. Alternative strategies may call for more staff, more equipment, more space, additional spending or a reduction in workload. After discussion with departmental staff of the options available the OR specialist may choose to use observations of the department at work to construct a mathematical model to be run as a computer simulation of the operation. Various changes to the model will then be made to represent the effect of, say, additional work or more effective equipment or changes in the work arrival pattern. The model simulation will show the likely result of different decisions. Although the most effective solution may be the most expensive, the model data will be used to support its application and will in turn also show that cheaper solutions will be less effective.

Thus far, OR has been applied to many organisational problems in health care and has much more to contribute. The use of queueing theory is particularly appropriate as there are many 'bottle-necks' in the process of health care and they are not all removed by simply increasing any single type of provision—throwing money at problems—which may merely transfer the bottle-neck elsewhere in the system. Some successful and fairly early work using OR techniques was carried out by Barber and Abbott at the London Hospital. It is no surprise that they state:

> The most successful work ... has always been done when potential users of the work participate actively in the technical aspects, contributing new ideas and suggestions for further studies and different types of data analysis as the work develops. Without active cooperation of this type, it is rarely possible to obtain vital operational data, to make recommendations or to attempt their implementation.'

Since a recommendation for prescriptive change may follow an OR analysis of a department or function, staff must participate in and contribute to the study in order to increase their 'stakeholding' in and their commitment to, the final outcome. Thus, as with the OD and the O and M workers, the OR specialist should be invited to participate in the analysis of organisational problems and contribute to their solution rather than to prescribe one *ex parte*.

Project Management

A particular technique in the OR repertoire suitable for project management is that of Network Analysis. This was developed to control the Polaris nuclear submarine project in the 1950s. It is appropriate where there are several operations and tasks that are dependent upon each other and where there are several sequences of dependent operations. This is typically illustrated by the management of building construction and is also applicable to the selection, purchase, installation and commissioning of a new piece of equipment such as a computer system or scanner or the transfer of a working department between different locations with minimal loss of service. In such projects where some activities have to be completed before others can begin the effect on the entire project of delay in a single activity is difficult to quantify. Sometimes the delay will be absorbed and at others an increase in total project time will occur. Network analysis will illustrate diagrammatically the interdependence of each component and show which sequences of activities are crucial for timely project management and where most acute attention must be focused to control outcome. This aspect is known as Critical Path Analysis. Furthermore, the amount of 'slack' in the non-critical pathways is quantified and this gives the manager a better perspective of the entire project.

However, the duration of every activity cannot always be precisely known and so it is possible, using probability theory, to include optimistic, pessimistic and the most likely duration time for each activity in the project and to forecast a range of outcomes depending on a combination of delays. Where the probability is high of an activity being delayed, particular attention can be given in advance to reduce that delay and to complete the project on time. This approach is known as Project Evaluation and Review Technique (PERT) and is applicable both before and during the project. It may also be combined with estimates of expenditure (COST-PERT) so that financial monitoring may form part of the control mechanism. From the network we may build up information not only regarding the order in which tasks are to be completed but also of the costs. Different skills may be required at different stages so that the direct starring costs will vary from activity to activity as will the materials and other non-staffing expenditure. The daily total costs of the project, therefore, are the sum of each parallel activity. By displaying these totals as part of a bar chart, or Gantt chart, as this is sometimes known, a manager is able to see at a glance exactly what should be occurring, together with the expected costs thereof. While the immediate consequences of sudden unplanned changes may be readily understood their effect on the remainder of the project and its running time will require calculation. Fortunately computer programs are available to run network analysis, to determine the critical path, to monitor COST-PERT and to provide updated information in response to changes. However, it is the manager who must act to keep the project on course and control the outcome by reference to the plan.

Budgetary Control

As a control instrument the budget is most appropriately

managed also by the use of a computer. 1'he daily expenditure incurred by undertaking work may be compared against the budgeted amount. The variance may be analysed, for example, by running mean calculation in order to smooth out daily fluctuations. By this means significant trends are identified. This analysis can be as detailed as required, once all the work of the department is monitored by the computer and the cost of each separate operation has been calculated and incorporated in the computer software. By analysing expenditure at sub-cost centre level, sensitive control information can be obtained given an adequate computer system. For large diagnostic clinical service and therapeutic departments investment in comprehensive computerized systems is almost a prerequisite for successful data collection.

In the private sector expenditure is substituted with profitability and each department or each section may be required to make a specified daily contribution to profit. It seems important to emphasize that the budget is employed as a control, whether in terms of expenditure or profit, because it is, or can be, a sensitive indicator and not because money is more important than the people needing care. Of course financial control is important in its own right and in this respect each general manager will have financial targets to meet. However, we have previously emphasized that quality of care requires to be agreed in the target-setting process and budgetary control should be applied to both the quality and quantity of work in each section of the health services. The obverse of implied prescriptive controls mediated through the application of such techniques as work study, operational research and budgetary control may be summarized in a single word—motivation. While such control mechanisms may be appropriately incorporated into organisational policy and plans, the effectiveness of their operation will depend upon the attitude adopted by staff. It could be argued that 'to motivate' is a managerial function and prerogative. However, we prefer to regard motivation as shared responsibility and dependent for its success on a variety of organisational and behavioural factors. Some of the many complexities of human interaction in the workplace are usefully discussed by Anthony and Fox among many other writers. From some of their work we conclude that organisationally effective motivation arises first in the mind of individual workers, is shared by fellow-workers and is congruent to enterprise objectives. Because such a state of mind does not always arise naturally, self-interest and group self-interest being potent forces within all organisations, 'motivation' has sometimes come to be regarded as a form of control which may be actively pursued by management in spite of "unhelpful' structural, organisational or behavioural impositions that militate against self-interest and harmony at work. Clearly, for self-motivation to develop, 'environmental' problems need to be resolved and individuals need to be able to have their needs met within the organisation. Some of the current problems associated with morale, motivation and management of paramedical and diagnostic service department staff in the NHS can be accounted for in these terms.

Management by Objectives (MBO)

The term 'Management by Objectives', MBO, was first introduced by Drucker to describe the process of self-control at work as opposed to managerial imposition. While each member of an enterprise contributes something different, says Drucker, their efforts must all contribute towards a common goal. Far from any notion of anarchy, Drucker argues that where individuals and managers are encouraged and assisted to set their own objectives, which must contribute to those of the organisation, their motivation will be strong and of the self-generating variety and their methods used to achieve objectives are more likely to be innovative, bold and efficient.

The principles of MBO elucidated by Drucker are that objectives should be specific and emphasize team work and should maximize individual and group contribution to enterprise objectives. Record-keeping should be confined to those records needed to complete each task—a reduction in the power of the bureaucratic process—and that the whole business should be characterized by a regular, upward communication by workers who would set their own objectives in consultation and by agreement with their managers. Drucker also drew attention to the problems of the role of the professional in organisations. Their work often militated against overall objectives in the name of the maintenance of professional standards, or by doing the 'best possible job' even when this was not called for in the corporate plan. This, he said, caused a 'misdirection' of vital resources.

A great deal of job satisfaction appears to be derived from operating as a 'professional' in the NHS and for management merely to discount or deny this source can only lead to lower morale and its associated problems. However, in MBO there lies a principle by which to involve many professionals, both medical and paramedical staff, in the objective-setting and decision-making process and in a transposition from organisational to self-control in management. It could be argued that while participation in setting objectives might well increase satisfaction, it need not necessarily lead to greater performance, but that is to beg the nature of the objectives themselves. MBO is characterized not only by the joint setting of rather difficult but realistic goals but also by a continual system of appraisal which involves giving feedback as to progress. Moreover, Cooper and Makin see MBO to be often associated with some incentive scheme, usually involving a whole package of changes. Locke, on the other hand, believes that it is the act of setting goals and striving to achieve them that motivates; the incentives and rewards he discounts as motivating factors. The choice of emphasis is perhaps governed by cultural forces, but the feedback and mutuality of MBO appear to meet a need in the managerial repertoire of the NHS. If we agreed with Anderson and Barnett that commitment, not compliance, and competence are the keys to improving staff effectiveness at work then managerial strategy is wisely aimed at obtaining and improving such commitment from, and competence of, its workers rather than merely obtaining their compliance. One of the principal ways this may be achieved is through an appropriate staff appraisal system.

Performance Appraisal

Management by objectives with regular feedback to the individual may be conveniently incorporated into a system of performance appraisal. Individual performance appraisal is regarded by Fletcher and Williams as having been one of the great growth industries of the 1960s and early 1970s. The aetiology, however, lies somewhere in the early 1900s, and early versions frequently adopted a judgemental style which was associated with 'personality' rather than 'performance'. As Fletcher observed, such appraisals were frequently difficult to relate in any very direct or constructive way to the job itself, tending to elicit defensive reactions where criticisms are given or implied. Even today, appraisal is associated by many with legalized criticism and an opportunity to learn from the manager about personal inadequacies.

Worse than this, because the term appraisal implies the making of a judgement, it may also be associated with disciplinary procedure being seen very clearly as a threat rather than an opportunity and as a process that emphasizes weaknesses, faults and subordination rather than strength, success and co-worker status. If appraisees are sceptical of its value, appraisers are equally reluctant to appraise. 'Mock' routinisation is often to be found where appraisals 'decay into routine form-filling, managers sometimes copying what they wrote the previous year'. Much of this unfortunate attitude is due to the fact that appraisal is widely seen mainly as a managerial prerogative, the manager merely legitimizing the continuing informal staff appraisal that is carried on *ex parte* in most organisations. In this informal system there is no opportunity for the appraisee to contribute and so the outcome is typically based on the manager's perceptions alone. Moreover, no records are kept; there is therefore no method of discovery and therefore no possibility of an appeal. Merely to formalize such a process, argues McGregor, means that managers are pushed unwillingly into a judicial role when formally appraising staff; not only are they obliged to make value judgements (playing God) for which they are unqualified but they must then see results of their judgements translated into organisational decisions which affect the lives and welfare of their staff, many of whom are likely to be closely related to them in the working situation.

Unilateral 'merit rating' of staff is emphatically not performance appraisal in the sense in which we understand the term. What we advocate here is, first, a system where standards, and the resources and support required to achieve those standards, will be mutually agreed between appraiser and appraisee and in which process there is a requisite bi-directional information flow that genuinely reflects the interdependence of both participants in the appraisal process. Second, a system which looks for, and rewards and builds on strengths rather than weaknesses and, third, a system that helps rather than punishes weaknesses and at the same time sets moderately difficult but attainable goals as in'centives.

Who Should Evaluate Performance?

Although it is possible to employ an appraisal specialist or to regard appraisal as a personnel function, the authors regard individual performance appraisal as a function of line management, with an equal 'stakeholding' and participation by the appraisee. The greater the commitment of both, the less threatening and ritualized the appraisal process will become. Clearly such involvement must include an element of self-review, and there is no certainty that both parties will sufficiently concur to reach agreement. Incongruence between the results of self-appraisal and those of management have tended to indicate lenience on the part of the self-appraiser, particularly when making comparisons with other workers. In general the appraisee is likely to have expectations of a more favourable outcome of the appraisal process than the appraiser. Reflection of this fact may go some way to explain the widely encountered negative attitude both toward the appraisal process as traditionally practised in Western industrial society and to the reception of criticism.

Thornton has shown that lenience in self-appraisal is also contex-tually dependent to some extent, being generally greater, for example, when the appraisal is directly related to pay. However, where the individual is asked to assess different aspects of his/her job performance relative to one another rather than against those of peers, research evidence indicates that subordinates' judgements are more discriminating than those of their superiors and that appraisals based on such self-assessment can be extremely effective.

Fletcher concurs, believing that 'such appraisals become more development centred, concentrating on the remedying of (relative) weakness and capitalizing on strength. The role that the subordinate has played in identifying these increases his or her willingness to implement action arising out of them.' While it is management's responsibility to conduct the appraisal process the manner of doing so and the participative role of the appraisee are crucial to its outcome. In a recent survey of nurse appraisals, Anderson and Barnett reported that the majority of survey participants indicated positive links between the appraisal interview and motivation, stating that, on the whole, they felt encouraged at the end of the interview. Other characteristics of these appraisals were that a majority of nurses found their appraiser supportive during the interview and that they enjoyed considerable freedom in putting forward and discussing their ideas and feelings at the appraisal interview. Appraisal then, is necessarily a shared activity.

Who Should be Evaluated?

Although the use of appraisal has for some time been mainly confined. to managerial staff and most particularly in large sector companies, Gill has shown that the few schemes for clerical/secretarial staff have been introduced more recently implying a growth in the use of appraisal with non-managerial staff. The low numbers of shop-floor workers appraised may be mainly due to trade union resistance to 'merit-rating'—a *de facto* shop-floor word for appraisal—and individual pay rates: a link always disfavoured by the unions who traditionally advocate collective bargaining. Promotion on the shop-floor still tends to be based on length of service. As with government-inspired attempts to introduce regular classroom assessments for teachers which have encountered union resistance, so the introduction of performance appraisal for some NHS workers will effect a cultural change and departure from established norms and, particularly if ultimately linked to pay, will tend to disenfranchize the trade unions as the principal staff-side negotiator of employer/employee relations. We discuss performance-related pay below. Meanwhile there appears to be no valid reason other than one of practicability why there should not be established an appraisal scheme for all or any grade of worker provided such schemes are designed to meet specific needs and requirements, are participative in style and benefit both the worker and the organisation.

What Kinds of Evaluations Should be Made?

Randell et al. categorize the many stated purposes of appraisal into three groups: Reward reviews: pay, power, status, freedom, self-fulfilment, i.e. benefits derived from the organisation. Performance reviews: assessment and improvement of individual performance and thereby that of the organisation. Potential reviews: predicting the type of work the individual will be capable of doing in the future and how long he/she will take to achieve this, together with the resources, training requirements and so on.

Reward Reciews

The bonus schemes and merit-rating approaches of scientific management represent the earliest formal appraisal practice. It was the inadequacy of these systems that led to a re-orientation of appraisal away from the reward reviews and towards a developmental approach. It would seem that the particular difficulties that were encountered with reward reviews revolved around the problems associated with the prerequisite measurement of individual job performance.

At the present time, the national salary structure and conditions of service for most NHS workers are set by the Whitley Councils, and effectively preclude the immediate employer from using discretionary awards to increase the pecuniary income of satisfactory employees. Must Whitley suffer the same fate as Burnham—the national negotiating body for the teachers—before reward reviews can be introduced? An alternative has been to seek an upgrading for the staff one wishes to reward and retain, particularly as a means of compensation for relatively low pay rates at basic grade level in a disadvantaged public sector. As for non-pecuniary awards, power status, privilege etc., these also tend to accompany grading: a consequence of the NHS bureaucratic infrastructure.

Potential Reviews

For many reasons there appears to be a predilection for the developmental approach to appraisal rather than for reward reviews or performance assessment. Of course, emphasis placed on the identification of potential and staff development circumvents the difficulties inherent in the other aspects of appraisal.

By placing emphasis on the future, current performance can be either partially discounted or considered solely in terms of personal development with corresponding de-emphasis on the attainment of organisational targets. This is also more comfortable for the manager as his/her responsibility for the appraisee's current performance is also not so critically examined. Apart from conflict avoidance, a further reason for this emphasis is that many NHS professional groups have highly developed expectations of personal and occupational group role development. They consequently maintain upward pressure on resources for further training, course and conference attendance and special work experience that will equip them for the future. Furthermore, many posts which carry heavy responsibility for work output and for which the organisation rightly expects total commitment are still regarded by many workers as post-basic 'stepping-stones' in personal career advancement. This is not to imply that in-work training courses are not wholly justified in the context of a continuously advancing medical science but it does help to explain the greater readiness of managers and staff alike to consider, preferentially, this aspect of the use of appraisal. Indeed, appetite for further study and personal advancement is likely to be a naturally occurring criterion in the appraisal of paramedical staff.

Performance Reviews

Although the purpose of appraisal schemes varies considerably, they are usually all regarded as serving organisational goals. However, Fletcher emphasizes that the appraisee also has needs and his/her expectations of appraisal may well include:

- the need to obtain feedback
- the reduction of uncertainty
- the influencing of career decisions, promotion, pay, etc.
- the seeking of advice and guidance.

Such needs may be expected to manifest themselves during the appraisal process, says Fletcher, and we would add that they raise the appraisee to a position of equal status with the appraiser in terms of the appraisal process. That is to say that each should be given the same preparation time, the same access to information, to records and to training to enable them to contribute equally in spite of the power differential that may exist between them. This balance is important. If we accept with Jones and Rogers that the 'prime purpose of appraisal is to improve individual or work group performance', then we are bound to consider that we may eventually suffer frustration of purpose. Edwards has argued that in due course the potential for progress in improvements in performance will become exhausted. This point, however, can be made the subject of negotiation as part of the appraisal. Considering the importance of the status of the appraisee, the legitimacy of the manager's right to appraise needs to be addressed. There are two aspects of this matter. First, in terms of legislation, particularly the Equal Opportunities law and subsequent case-law interpretation thereof, the manager's right to appraise is constrained by the requirement of job-relatedness. This is already established in the United States, although judicial status for appraisal forms is not yet conferred in the United Kingdom.

Second, there is the more fundamental issue of the duties and obligations implied by the contract of employment. We believe that the expressed and implied terms of the employment contract, together with the degree of flexibility, usually incorporated therein, generally gives sanction to the well-prepared, job-related appraisal scheme. For example: 'Employers have a duty to cooperate with the employee, i.e. they must not destroy the mutual trust and confidence upon which cooperation is built. 'Employers must employ competent and safe fellow workers.

'Employees have a duty to cooperate with the employer, the duty of fidelity and to carry out lawful and reasonable instructions.'Beyond contractual considerations lies the undercurrent of diffuse obligations so frequently invoked by many employers and accepted by many employees that mean that the claims of the employer are not necessarily discounted but are viewed in a broader perspective. It is this perspective that can not only legitimize the appraisal process but establish it as a means of organisational learning, of personal growth and development for both appraiser and appraisee as well as a means by which to optimize efficiency and effectiveness throughout the organisation.

For What Purpose Should Evaluations be Made?

Many writers advise that each appraisal system should have one purpose only and that to mix reward reviews, say, with development of performance assessment is to introduce, unnecessarily, potential conflict, stress and misdirection of purpose into the system. Of course, some degree of overlap is unavoidable but in general we see the primary purpose of performance appraisal in the NHS as being:

- To bring about and maintain satisfactory performance on the part of individual employees by monitoring their effectiveness on the job and by encouraging them to comment on the support of managers to which their effectiveness is related.
- To encourage and facilitate personal growth and development of all those involved in the appraisal process.
- To provide an additional and formal means of organisational learning.

It is clear that in order to meet these objectives certain prerequisites must be obtained, i.e.:

- The clear and unequivocal commitment on the part of both appraiser and appraisee to the appraisal process. This naturally implies a similar organisational commitment if rituals, archaic processes and 'mock' bureaucracy are to be avoided.
- The subsumption of legitimate individual goals with those of the organisation.
- The establishment of an effective system of two-way communication integral to the appraisal process.
- The agreement of all concerned as to the dimensions

of the appraisal system. This will involve the identification of criteria, personal constructs, prejudices, etc., that managers and employees alike carry with them.

- The identification of training needs for all concerned.
- The development of appraisal forms (the Appraisal Instrument of Latham and Wexley), and their validation.
- The on-going evaluation of the scheme to maintain effectiveness particularly with respect to the organisational changes which may be anticipated as a result of the use of performance appraisal.

There is no single system of appraisal which will suit all circumstances or groups of workers, even in the Health Service, or all organisations. In fact Randell et al. argue for appraisal schemes that not only have single objectives but that are compatible with the organisational culture *at a given time* and that may change to meet changing needs of both the organisation and the individuals who comprise it. Appraisal models successfully used for nurses, therefore, may be inappropriate for pharmacists, porters or MLSOs. However, by adopting an MBO approach, appraisal may focus less on determining a rating or assessment of past individual performance and more on achievement of agreed future objectives and the resources required to attain them. Such an approach requires job analysis, a goal-oriented job description, a clear understanding of what is required of each individual by the manager, participation by the employee and the development of a dialogue in the appraisal interview. Moreover, each appraisal requires to be individualized to meet the needs of each employee and his or her particular circumstances at work.

'If the appraisal is going to be accepted by an employee

whose performance is under review he must *see* that full account is taken of those factors within his work situation which he believes restrict or inhibit his personal contributions', says M.R. Williams. In other words, the appraisal must be of the 'individual-in-the-job; not merely of the individual himself. On the appraisal form, therefore, may be written agreed targets to be achieved by the appraisee, together with the support and resources deemed to be required from the manager and the expected date of attainment. Both participants have a copy of the form which may also record other points raised by either person. Because this approach calls for negotiating skills, the training requirement for this type of scheme is substantial. It is far easier to award workers, say, an A or B for past performance than to negotiate with them a change in working practice. It cannot be assumed that many NHS managers possess these skills, therefore training with practice is mandatory before embarking on this exercise.

This requires a willingness to 'have a go' and to be prepared to make mistakes in order to learn. 'While knowledge can be got through books', say Stewart and Stewart, 'skills must be acquired through practice with feedback, the trainee actually performing the task to be learned rather than passively watching or absorbing information.'Responsiveness to the training programme is therefore an important criterion when deciding who is able to conduct appraisals. Since this is a line management function it is reasonable that this should become incorporated into the criteria for management appointments. The aim of appraisal, then, is to improve managerial control by improving self-direction of all workers. After appropriate research, schemes should be developed specifically to meet particular organisational requirements and be appropriate for particular groups of staff. There are many books specifically written to assist in this matter and the authors recommend particularly those of Fletcher and Williams,Stewart and Stewart and Randell et al. These may be studied as an introduction to the implementation of appraisal schemes. However, the authors believe that the most important ingredient for success is the commitment of time. Anderson and Barnett report that in their study, 52% of nurse managers stated that they devoted between a half and one hour to interview preparation for each member of their staff, while 31 % indicated they spent between one and two hours in preparation for each interview. By contrast the length of the appraisal interviews was often quite short, 65% of the interviews were of less than 40 minutes duration and 33%, less than 25 minutes. Anderson and Barnett quote the results of a national survey by Longwhich showed that most appraisal interviews of managerial staff last for between one and two hours, and conclude that 'it seems most unlikely that meaningful, in-depth discussion reviewing a whole year's work and planning for the year ahead could take place in such a short time' (i.e. less than 25 minutes). From this we conclude that the benefits of performance appraisal will reflect the commitment it receives.

Performance-Related Pay (PRP)

At first sight it would seem a short step to take from individual performance review to performance-related pay. On reflection, the introduction of PRP is perhaps the biggest cultural shock to the system so far. Low pay in the NHS is either regarded as the *sine qua non* of dedicated professionalism or as a social obscenity. The truth, we suspect, is that pay and dedication are only very weakly related, if at all, and that most health workers across a wide range of occupations choose to work in health care because they want to. It follows that although people want to be rewarded and will work harder if they are, there is a point beyond which pecuniary reward will have rapidly diminishing returns. On the other hand, the recognition, goal-setting and positive feedback likely to arise from a good appraisal scheme or individual performance review as it is known, is far more likely to be highly motivating provided there is an adequate and realistic level of basic pay and reasonable working conditions already in place on which to build. By introducing PRP only at the top of the organisation the management board run the risk of creating a good deal of bad feeling. The success of general managers depends wholly upon the support and efficiency of those below actually to attain organisational goals and reach targets—targets that may well have been negotiated with those subordinate staff. They too will demand their reward, as will their subordinates, and so on throughout the organisation.

The introduction of PRP will not be helped by the fact that most of the original targets will need to be financial savings of various kinds. It is obvious that part of such savings will be used to 'reward' the general managers themselves while many sub-unit staff will be asked to improve their service with less resources and no personal financial reward. If savings are required to be made then it is the general manager's task to make them and the question has to be asked why additional money is payable to general managers only, rather than to any other health workers for doing the job for which they were engaged? The truth is that PRP is not an appropriate system for rewarding professional staff. If it were, the winners under PRP would enjoy their bonuses at the expense of the losers since little extra income can be generated in the NHS by extra effort and efficiency. This is not a scenario that will enhance morale. PRP is likely to work against the implementation of performance appraisal since such institutionalized inequalities in the system will inhibit cooperation. The whole idea is reminiscent of Herzberg's description 'jumping for the jellybeans'. After a while larger and larger quantities of beans are required in order to elicit the required response! Wall, in a penetrating article, asks 'who sets the objectives for PRP?' A further question relates to their assessment. Since the scheme is 'geared to rewarding quantifiable achievement', how will the called-for improvements in service quality be rewarded? How will such improvements be assessed and how directly responsible will general managers be deemed to be for these improvements? Organisational control is about the management of the entire enterprise rather than a compromise between relative success in some parts supporting relative failure in others. PRP does not seem to use an appropriate mechanism of control in health care generally, or the NHS in particular. The stick and the carrot both belong to the management of donkeys; we doubt they have anything that is positive to contribute to patient well-being.

Personnel Policies and Procedures

Finally, organisations need to maintain control even when things go wrong and break down. The personnel department will develop policies covering the legal obligations of the organisation as an employer. These will include such matters as equal opportunities, employment, health and safety, disciplinary and grievance procedures. For an employee to declare a grievance or for a manager to resort to disciplinary procedure, it should not necessarily mean that the individuals involved are somehow emotionally 'lost' to the organisation and that their loyalty will be irreparably damaged. However, if skills training in appraisal procedure is poorly developed the same holds for disciplinary and grievance procedures, the traditional view being that these are the province of the personnel department. This is a misleading notion. Whereas the advice and assistance of personnel are indis-pensible, the responsibility in these matters always remains with the line manager who requires knowledge of the personnel policies of the organisation together with an understanding of current employment law. The manager also needs to possess the personal and social skills to carry out that policy swiftly, fairly and with equanimity. Small problems if handled in this way will usually be resolved with little recourse to formal proceedings. Left too long or mishandled they can grow into large, formal, expensive affairs taking an enormous time commitment to complete.

While the end process of disciplinary procedure is the termination of employment, the various steps in the process aim to provide opportunity for improved performance. Any disciplinary action should normally be accompanied by appropriate retraining and review. It is important that performance appraisal and discipline are kept apart. There may be times when this is not possible but as a general rule such an association in the minds of staff will not help either process. A further problem may arise when managers attempt to use counselling as part of these interactive processes with staff. It may be thought that as long as the subject matter is work-related, counselling may take place. Milne, has drawn a clear distinction between coaching, using counselling skills and counselling. The manager, because of his/her organisational role, is at a major disadvantage as a counsellor. It is often impossible and inappropriate for managers to be non-judgemental and non-directive and it is improper for them to agree to keep confidences that may conflict with their work role as employers. As a personal problem at work unfolds, frequently issues are revealed that may be more appropriately addressed by referral to a counsellor who is not directly employed by the organisation and who reports to no-one. Some authorities retain such people who are available via the personnel or occupational health departments. The use of counselling skills, on the other hand, may indeed be valuable in many managerial activities. The development of these skills requires training and we hope to see such investment in NHS staff as the new NHS Training Authority exerts its influence at district level and beyond.To control is a managerial prerogative but it is exercised effectively with the consent of staff and must therefore be appropriate to their needs. Such control requires skill and such skills must be acquired through practice. The current emphasis on skills training seeks to improve the quality of managerial performance in this respect and by so doing, in part, raises the quality of health care and thereby ultimately contributes to the improvement of the health of our nation.

6

Towards Fixing Heath Education & Management Systems and Services

EVALUATION AND MANAGEMENT SERVICES FOR INPATIENT VISITS

One of the most important aims of developing new evaluation and management codes was to make the coding for visits for hospitalized patients more rational. The descriptions of visits and the allocation of both "time" and "work" were changed. The guiding principle now is documentation. Medicare carriers will request documentation of activity, and it is strongly advised that all consultations and admissions be dictated. In daily progress notes, physicians should write the date, the time of the progress note, and their subspecialty designation (1/4/92, 1330, Rheumatology), and then the body of the progress note.

Hospital visits can be separated into two broad groups: (1) visits for which the physician is the primary attending; and (2) visits for which the physician is the consultant. A detailed explanation of office consultations. In this chapter, it is important to understand that consultations are regarded differently in the hospital than in the office. The most important difference is that the follow-up consultation codes are available for hospitalized patients but not for office patients.

Visits for which the rheumatologist is the primary attending will be addressed first. The relevant CPT codes are divided into initial observation care, initial hospital care and subsequent hospital care with three levels of services. Descriptions for each level of service in this chapter are taken from the AMA CPT manual for definitions of the levels of E/M services. Each level of service is followed by a patient encounter example. Some of the patient encounter examples have been validated by the AMA; however, many of the examples have not been validated and are subject to change. Only those examples labeled "AMA/CPT validated example" have gone through the AMA validation process.

INITIAL OBSERVATION CARE: NEW OR ESTABLISHED PATIENT

Initial observation care codes (99218-99220) are used to report the first encounter by the supervising physician with the patient when designated as "observation status." This refers to the initiation of observation status, supervision of the care plan for observation and performance of periodic assessments. It is not necessary that the hospital have a designated area in which observation services are performed. If such an area does exist in a hospital (as a separate unit in the hospital, in the emergency department, etc.), these codes are to be used if the patient is placed there.

Only the supervising physician admitting the patient to "observation status" may use these codes. If a consultation is requested by this admitting physician, the consulting physician would use outpatient consultation codes (99241-99245).

If a patient is seen in "observation status" and admitted to the hospital the same day, an initial hospital care code (99221-99223), which includes the work of the combined E/

M services, should be used. If a patient is seen in "observation status" today and admitted to the hospital tomorrow, an initial observation care code (99218-99220) should be used to bill for today's services, and an initial hospital care code (99221-99223) should be used for tomorrow's services.

When "observation status" is initiated in the course of an encounter in another site of service (e.g., hospital emergency department, physician's office or nursing facility) an initial observation care code, which includes the work of the combined E/M services, should be used. E/M services on the same date provided in sites that are related to initiating "observation status" should not be reported separately.

Initial observation care codes may not be used for post-operative recovery if the procedure is considered part of a global surgical procedure. Also note, these codes apply to all E/M services that are provided on the same day of patient admission to "observation status."

An initial history and physical should be performed on each patient admitted to "observation status." This is true even if the admitting physician also performed a history and physical in the hospital emergency department. Physicians should note the date and time of the history and physical to make it clear to auditors that the physical was performed after the patient was admitted to "observation status."

Initial observation care, per day, for the evaluation and management of a patient which requires the following three key components:

1. A detailed or comprehensive history
2. A detailed or comprehensive examination
3. Medical decision making that is straightforward or of low complexity

Counseling and/or coordination of care with other providers or agencies are provided consistent with the nature of the problem(s) and the patient's and/or family's needs.

Usually, the problem(s) requiring admission to "observation status" are of low severity.

Initial observation care, per day, for the evaluation and management of a patient which requires the following three key components:

1. A comprehensive history
2. A comprehensive examination
3. Medical decision making of moderate complexity

Counseling and/or coordination of care with other providers or agencies are provided consistent with the nature of the problem(s) and the patient's and/or family's needs.

Usually, the problem(s) requiring admission to "observation status" are of moderate severity.

Initial observation care, per day, for the evaluation and management of a patient which requires the following three key components:

1. A comprehensive history
2. A comprehensive examination
3. Medical decision making of high complexity

Counseling and/or coordination of care with other providers or agencies are provided consistent with the nature of the problem(s) and the patient's and/or family's needs.

Usually, the problem(s) requiring admission to "observation status" are of high severity.

Observation Care Discharge Services

CPT code 99217 is to be used to report all services

provided to a patient on discharge from "observation status" if the discharge is on a day other than the initial date of "observation status." Discharge of a patient from "observation status" includes final examination of the patient, discussion of the hospital stay, instructions for continuing care and preparation of discharge records.

Observation Care Discharge Day Management

To report services to a patient designated as "observation status" who is discharged on the same date, use only the codes for initial observation services (99218-99220).

Initial Hospital Care:New or Established Patient

Most third party payors will not reimburse for more than one medical visit by the same provider per day. If a patient is seen in the office, and admitted to the hospital the same day, a single code must be assigned to the E/M services provided if they were for the same diagnosis. In such cases, billing the code for the initial hospital care should reflect the work of these combined services because, in general, initial hospital codes will provide the appropriate reimbursement for the services rendered since these codes assume time spent in reviewing radiographs and give credit for physician "floor time."

If the diagnosis is different for the E/M services provided on the same day, then two codes, one reflecting office service and the other reflecting admission service, are appropriate. Selection of the CPT and ICD-9-CM codes and subsequent documentation should indicate why the second visit was appropriate. *Note: For Medicare billing purposes, if an admission and office visit are performed on the same day, bill only the admission. If two hospital visits are billed on the same day, only one will be reimbursed unless the second one is for an emergency situation (e.g., the patient is admitted with a stable condition that becomes unstable later in the day). Medicare will consider payment for the second visit on a post-payment basis. Another alternative may be prolonged detention. Generally, codes are considered as services per day.*

When the patient is admitted to the hospital as an inpatient, in the course of an encounter in another site of service (e.g., hospital emergency department, observation status in a hospital, physician's office, nursing facility), all evaluation and management services provided by that physician in conjunction with that admission are considered part of the initial hospital care when performed on the same date as the admission. The inpatient care level of service reported by the admitting physician should include the services related to the admission he/she provided in the other sites of service as well as in the inpatient setting.

Evaluation and management services on the same date provided in sites other than the hospital that are related to the admission should *not* be reported separately.

CPT codes 99221-99233 are used to report the first hospital inpatient encounter with the patient by the admitting physician. (For initial inpatient encounters by physicians other than the admitting physician, see initial inpatient consultation codes 99251-99255 or subsequent hospital care codes 99231-99233).

Initial hospital care, per day, for the evaluation and management of a patient which requires the following three key components:

1. A detailed or comprehensive history
2. A detailed or comprehensive examination
3. Medical decision making that is straightforward or of low complexity

Counseling and/or coordination of care with other providers or agencies are provided consistent with the nature of the problem(s) and the patient's and/or family's needs. Usually, the problem(s) requiring admission are of low severity. Physicians typically spend 30 minutes at the bedside and on the patient's hospital floor or unit.

Examples

1. Hospital admission of a 27-year-old female with lupus nephritis for her first course of cytoxan therapy. The patient is well known to her physician, is a compliant patient and was seen in the office five days earlier. Results of lab tests are available at the time of admission.

2. AMA/CPT validated example: Initial hospital visit for a 62-year-old female with stable rheumatoid arthritis, admitted for total joint replacement.

Initial hospital care, per day, for the evaluation and management of a patient, which requires the following three key components:

1. A comprehensive history
2. A comprehensive examination
3. Medical decision making of moderate severity

Counseling and/or coordination of care with other providers or agencies are provided consistent with the nature of the problem(s) and the patient's and/or family's needs.

Usually, the problem(s) requiring admission are of moderate severity. Physicians typically spend 50 minutes at the bedside and on the patient's hospital floor or unit.

Example

1. Hospital admission of a 19-year-old female with fever, rash and an acute monoarthritis. Comprehensive history,

review of systems, social history and examination performed. Appropriate cultures, radiographs and laboratory ordered. Joint aspiration performed. Antibiotics instituted for presumed gonococcal arthritis. Patient education as to etiology of illness.

A hospital visit performed by the same physician on the day of a minor starred (*) surgical procedure such as arthrocentesis may be reported separately if the patient's condition required a significant, separately identifiable E/ M service above and beyond the usual preoperative and postoperative care associated with the procedure. This event may be reported by adding the modifier "-25" to the appropriate hospital visit code (or indicated by 09925), in addition to coding for the procedure. Note: HCFA does not recognize starred procedures. The procedures eligible for a "-25" modifier are those with zero or 10 post-operative days.

Initial hospital care, per day, for the evaluation and management of a patient, which requires the following three key components:

1. A comprehensive history
2. A comprehensive examination
3. Medical decision making of high complexity

Counseling and/or coordination of care with other providers or agencies are provided consistent with the nature of the problem(s) and the patient's and/or family's needs.

Usually, the problem(s) requiring admission are of high severity. Physicians typically spend 70 minutes at the bedside and on the patient's hospital floor or unit.

Examples

1. Hospital admission for a 42-year-old woman with rapidly progressive scleroderma, malignant hypertension,

digital infarcts and renal failure. Comprehensive history and physical examination performed. Diagnostic tests ordered. Antihypertensive therapy instituted. Other consultants contacted. Prognosis discussed with patient and family.

2. AMA/CPT validated example: Initial hospital visit for a 42-year-old female with rapidly progressing scleroderma, malignant hypertension, digital infarcts and oligourea.

3. Hospital admission for a 53-year-old female with previous breast cancer (without clinical evidence of recurrence), hypothyroidism, and Stage 2, Class 2 rheumatoid arthritis. Patient is admitted because of the development of mononeuritis multiplex in three extremities and painful purpura over the left lower leg. Comprehensive history and physical examination are performed. Diagnostic studies are ordered, detailed management orders are written and the dose of intravenous cytoxan is calculated and ordered, along with detailed instructions for its administration. The diagnosis and treatment are discussed with the patient's daughter and son-in-law.

If this visit required the rheumatologist to provide unusually intense services for a severely ill patient, the codes 99356-99357 may be used to describe prolonged evaluation and management services in the inpatient setting requiring direct (face-to-face) patient contact beyond the usual service. Prolonged service of less than 30 minutes total duration cannot be reported separately. For guidelines on using prolonged services codes (99354-99357).

4. AMA/CPT validated example: Initial hospital visit for a 35-year-old female with severe systemic lupus erythematosus on corticosteroid and cyclophosphamide, with new onset of fever, chills, rash and chest pain.

5. AMA/CPT validated example: Initial hospital visit for a 40-year-old female with anatomical stage 3, ARA functional class 3 rheumatoid arthritis on methotrexate, corticosteroid and nonsteroidal anti-inflammatory drugs. Patient presents with severe arthritis flare, new oral ulcers, abdominal pain and leukopenia.

Subsequent Hospital Care

Coding for subsequent hospital care should reflect the level and intensity of service required for the individual patient on a particular day. Codes for daily care may vary depending on the possible development of new problems or worsening of existing problems. These codes are meant to be used for all care provided on a given day. If the rheumatologist visits or sees a hospital inpatient more than once a day, all such encounters and all care rendered for the patient on that day should be combined in one level of service code (For payment purposes, Medicare will combine both the office and admission services into a single hospital visit. The only time it will not is if the later visit is for emergency purposes — then it will only pay on a post payment basis). The exceptions are a return visit for complications constituting critical care or for a second distinct problem which requires a different ICD-9-CM code. In the former case, both a hospital care code (for non-critical care) and a critical care code should be used with supporting documentation to show that both services were necessary.

All levels of subsequent hospital care include reviewing the medical record and reviewing the results of diagnostic studies and changes in the patient's status (e.g., change in history, physical condition and response to management) since the last assessment by the physician.

Subsequent hospital care, per day, for the evaluation

and management of a patient, which requires at least two of the following three key components:

1. A problem focused interval history
2. A problem focused examination
3. Medical decision making that is straightforward or of low complexity

Counseling and/or coordination of care with other providers or agencies are provided consistent with the nature of the problem(s) and the patient's and/or family's needs.

Usually the patient is stable, recovering or improving. Physicians typically spend 15 minutes at the bedside and on the patient's hospital floor or unit.

Examples

1. Follow-up hospital visit for a 55-year-old female with rheumatoid arthritis, three days following an uncomplicated joint replacement. Patient's general medical care is being managed by her internist. Brief examination and chart review completed. Medications adjusted accordingly.

2. AMA/CPT validated example: Subsequent hospital visit for a 55-year-old male with rheumatoid arthritis, two days following an uncomplicated joint replacement.

Subsequent hospital care, per day, for the evaluation and management of a patient, which requires at least two of the following three key components:

1. An expanded problem focused interval history
2. An expanded problem focused examination
3. Medical decision making of moderate complexity

Counseling and/or coordination of care with other providers or agencies are provided consistent with the nature of the problem(s) and the patient's and/or family's needs.

Usually, the patient is responding inadequately to therapy or has developed a minor complication. Physicians typically spend 25 minutes at the bedside and on the patient's hospital floor or unit.

Examples

1. Follow-up hospital visit for a 55-year-old female with rheumatoid arthritis, and three days of postoperative leg pain and swelling from total hip replacement. Patient's general medical care is being managed by the rheumatologist. She denies chest pain, shortness of breath or a flare of rheumatoid arthritis. Complete examination performed. Anticoagulant therapy instituted for presumed deep venous thrombosis. Venous study ordered. Rheumatologist discussed plan with the orthopedic surgeon.

2. Follow-up visit for an 85-year-old female with a recently dislocated total hip replacement who was admitted by the orthopedic surgeon for the replacement and who was seen by the rheumatologist after general anesthesia. She was again seen by the rheumatologist after she had returned to her room. On the second hospital day, she is slightly obtunded, and her short-term memory is impaired. Electrolytes, including magnesium level and CT scan, are ordered by the rheumatologist. Rheumatologist consulted with a neurologist after conferring with the orthopedic surgeon.

Subsequent hospital care, per day, for the evaluation and management of a patient, which requires at least two of the following three key components:

1. A detailed interval history
2. A detailed examination
3. Medical decision making of high complexity

Counseling and/or coordination of care with other

providers or agencies are provided consistent with the nature of the problem(s) and the patient's and/or family's needs.

Usually, the patient is unstable or has developed a significant complication or a significant new problem. Physicians typically spend 35 minutes at the bedside and on the patient's hospital floor or unit.

Examples

1. Follow-up hospital visit for a 25-year-old female with systemic lupus erythematosus, hypertension, fever and respiratory distress. Any medical complications are being managed by the rheumatologist. On the third hospital day, the patient developed purpuric skin lesions and renal failure. Detailed examination and chart review completed. Appropriate specific therapy instituted by the rheumatologist. Nephrology consultation obtained. Prognosis discussed with family members.

2. AMA/CPT validated example: Subsequent hospital visit for a 25-year-old female with hypertension and systemic lupus erythematosus, admitted for fever and respiratory distress. On the third hospital day, the patient presented with purpuric skin lesions and acute renal failure.

3. AMA/CPT validated example: Subsequent hospital visit for a 65-year-old female with rheumatoid arthritis (Stage 3, Class 3) admitted for urosepsis. On the third hospital day, chest pain, dyspnea and fever develop.

Hospital Discharge Services

The hospital discharge day management codes are to be used to report the total duration of time spent by a physician for final hospital discharge of a patient. The codes include, as appropriate, final examination of the patient, discussion of the hospital stay, even if the time spent by the physician on that date is not continuous. Instructions for continuing care are give to all relevant caregivers, and preparation of discharge records, prescriptions and referral forms is completed. The patient does not have to be seen, but services have to be provided on the date billed.

Hospital discharge day management, 30 minutes or less.

Hospital discharge day management, more than 30 minutes.

To report services for a patient who is admitted as an inpatient and discharged on the same day, use only the codes for initial hospital inpatient services (99221-99223). To report concurrent care services provided by a physician(s) other than the attending physician, use subsequent hospital care codes (99231-99233) on the day of discharge.

Hospital Consultations

In contrast with previous CPT coding practices, different codes are used for inpatient and outpatient consultations. The Harvard RBRVS study showed that inpatient work and overhead were quite different from outpatient work and overhead for consultations. Consequently, different descriptors are used for inpatient consultations.

Additionally, inpatient consultation codes provide for follow-up consultations, whereas outpatient consultation codes do not. *It is critical to note that outpatient consultation codes cannot be used for inpatients, and vice / versa.* Residents of nursing facilities qualify as inpatients under the initial and follow-up inpatient consultation codes.

Please refer to the definitions and guidelines for a consultation. Initial inpatient consultations have five levels of services while follow-up inpatient consultations have three levels of services. Each level of service is followed by a patient encounter example. These examples imply that the .rheumatology consultant communicates (orally or in written form) with the requesting physician about the patient work-up, differential diagnosis and potential treatment options. *Note: For Medicare billing purposes, a hospital inpatient consultation must be supported by a written request by the attending physician on the chart. Rules for out-of-hospital consults may vary. Check with your Medicare carrier.*

Initial Inpatient Consultations: New or Established Patient

The following codes are used to report physician consultations provided to hospital inpatients, residents of nursing facilities or patients in a partial hospital setting. Only one initial consultation should be reported by a consultant per admission. (For additional examples, please refer to the new patient office visit codes (99201-99205) or the outpatient consultation codes (99241-99245) with the addition of a request for a consultation in the hospital from another physician.)

Initial inpatient consultation for a new or established patient, which requires the following three key components:

1. A problem focused history
2. A problem focused examination
3. Straightforward medical decision making

Counseling and/or coordination of care with other providers or agencies are provided consistent with the nature of the problem(s) and the patient's and/or family's needs.

Usually, the presenting problem(s) are self limited or minor. Physicians typically spend 20 minutes at the bedside and on the patient's hospital floor or unit.

Initial inpatient consultation for a new or established patient, which requires the following three key components:

1. An expanded problem focused history
2. An expanded problem focused examination
3. Straightforward medical decision making

Counseling and/or coordination of care with other providers or agencies are provided consistent with the nature of the problem(s) and the patient's and/or family's needs.

Usually, the presenting problem(s) are of low severity. Physicians typically spend 40 minutes at the bedside and on the patient's hospital floor or unit.

Example

1. Hospital consultation for a 72-year-old male patient recovering from angioplasty who develops an acute bursitis of the left shoulder. The rheumatologist had seen the patient four years previously for an episode of pseudogout in the right knee. The patient is on anti-hypertensive and lipid-lowering drugs. He is afebrile and otherwise has made an uneventful recovery. Routine lab studies are unremarkable and an admission chest x-ray showed only mild cardiomegaly.

Initial inpatient consultation for a new or established patient which requires the following three key components:

1. A detailed history
2. A detailed examination
3. Medical decision making of low complexity

Counseling and/or coordination of care with other providers or agencies are provided consistent with the nature of the problem(s) and the patient's and/or family's needs.

Usually, the presenting problem(s) are of moderate

severity. Physicians typically spend 55 minutes at the bedside and on the patient's hospital floor or unit.

Examples

1. Hospital consultation for an obese female hospitalized for an endoscopic removal of her gallbladder. She is making an apparently uneventful recovery from a moderately difficult procedure. On the third hospital day (which was going to be her discharge day), she develops right podagra and pain in multiple joints. In addition to a bright red first toe, she has warmth and an effusion in her left knee. The rheumatologist is consulted. The family is present and is anxious about this complication; they remind the rheumatologist that the patient's brother was seen by the rheumatologist for gout. Records reviewed, x-rays ordered and knee aspirated, with fluid sent to the laboratory. Gout crystals found, and therapy initiated. The rheumatologist informs family that the patient will be seen the next day for review.

A hospital consultation performed by the same physician on the day of a minor starred (*) surgical procedure such as arthrocentesis may be reported separately if the patient's condition required a significant, separately identifiable E / M service above and beyond the usual preoperative and postoperative care associated with the procedure. This event may be reported by adding modifier "-25" to the appropriate hospital consultation code (or indicated by 09925), in addition to coding for the procedure. Note: HCFA does not recognize starred procedures. The procedures eligible for a "-25" modifier are those with zero or 10 post-operative days.

2. Hospital consultation requested by an internist who has admitted a 38-year-old postal worker with an episode of pneumonia. The patient is on his fourth day of antibiotics, and he is coughing less and has only a slight fever. His pleuritic chest pain has resolved, but he is still coughing

heavily. When he coughs or when he sits up for more than 15 or 20 minutes, he develops low back pain which radiates posteriorly down his left leg past the knee. A brother has had an unfortunate experience after back surgery, and the patient does not want surgery. The rheumatologist is consulted and a detailed history and examination are performed which show evidence of mild radiculopathy. The rheumatologist discussed the case with the patient and his wife and prescribed a course of therapy. The rheumatologist will follow jointly with the internist, who will manage the pneumonia.

Initial inpatient consultation for a new or established patient which requires the following three key components:

1. A comprehensive history
2. A comprehensive examination
3. Medical decision making of moderate complexity

Counseling and/or coordination of care with other providers or agencies are provided consistent with the nature of the problem(s) and the patient's and/or family's needs.

Usually the presenting problem(s) are of moderate to high severity. Physicians typically spend 80 minutes at the bedside and on the patient's hospital floor or unit.

Examples

1. Hospital consultation for a 68-year-old woman admitted for a six-month history of severe polyarthritis. The arthritis is unresponsive to initial therapy. The patient's family is present. Comprehensive history and musculoskeletal examination performed. Review of laboratory studies, chart and x-rays completed with patient and family, consistent with rheumatoid arthritis. Treatment options, drug toxicity, and long-term prognosis discussed with patient and family.

The addition of "second-line" antirheumatic therapy instituted and physical therapy consultation arranged.

2. AMA/CPT validated example: Initial inpatient consultation for 35-year-old female with fever, swollen joints and rash of one week duration.

Initial inpatient consultation for a new or established patient which requires the following three key components:

1. A comprehensive history
2. A comprehensive examination
3. Medical decision making of high complexity

Counseling and/or coordination of care with other providers or agencies are provided consistent with the nature of the problem(s) and the patient's and/or family's needs.

Usually the presenting problem(s) are of moderate to high severity. Physicians typically spend 110 minutes at the bedside and on the patient's hospital floor or unit.

Examples

1. Initial hospital consultation for a 22-year-old steroid-dependent woman with systemic lupus erythematosus, arthritis and glomerulonephritis. Patient is re-evaluated for loss of consciousness and chest pain. Comprehensive examination performed. Review of x-rays, cardiac echo cardiogram, laboratory studies and chart completed. Case discussed with patient and her nephrologist and cardiologist. Appropriate diagnostic studies ordered. Steroid dosage adjusted along with institution of anticoagulation.

2. Initial hospital consultation for a 6-year-old boy with one month of persistent fever, rash, joint pain, thrombocytopenia, abnormal liver tests and coagulopathy. Comprehensive examination performed. Laboratory tests

and copies of pertinent outpatient charts from the offices of six other involved physicians reviewed. Case discussed with other consultants, including infectious diseases, hematology and gastroenterology. The diagnosis of Still's Disease is considered likely. Appropriate specific therapy instituted, along with adjustments of other medications. Prognosis for Still's Disease was discussed with other family members.

Follow-Up Inpatient Consultations: Established Patient

The follow-up inpatient consultation codes are used for established hospital inpatient or nursing facility patients only. For consultative services provided in other settings, office or other outpatient consultations codes (99241-99245) should be reported.

Follow-up consultations are visits initiated by the rheumatology consultant to complete the initial consultation or subsequent consultative visits requested by the attending physician. According to the AMA CPT manual, a follow-up consultation includes monitoring progress, recommending management modifications or advising on a new plan of care in response to changes in the patient's status.

If the rheumatology consultant has assumed the care of the patient after initiating treatment at the initial consultation, then the codes for subsequent hospital care (CPT 99231-99233) should be used.

Follow-up inpatient consultation for an established patient which requires at least two of the following three key components:

1. A problem focused interval history
2. A problem focused examination
3. Medical decision making that is straightforward or of low complexity

Counseling and/or coordination of care with other providers or agencies are provided consistent with the nature of the problem(s) and the patient's and/or family's needs.

Usually, the patient is stable, recovering or improving. Physicians typically spend 10 minutes at the bedside and on the patient's hospital floor or unit.

Examples

1. AMA/CPT validated example: Follow-up inpatient consultation with a 67-year-old female, established patient, for review of diagnostic studies ordered at time of first contact.

This example would fit a rheumatologic patient with osteoarthritis.

2. Follow-up consultation for the female patient described in the example under CPT code 99253. The patient is feeling better. The podagra is gone and the knee feels only slightly warm. The surgeon wants to discharge the patient. The patient is scheduled to see the rheumatologist in one week.

Follow-up inpatient consultation for an established patient which requires at least two of the following three key components:

1. An expanded problem focused interval history
2. An expanded problem focused examination
3. Medical decision making of moderate complexity

Counseling and/or coordination of care with other providers or agencies are provided consistent with the nature of the problem(s) and the patient's and/or family's needs.

Usually the patient is responding inadequately to therapy or has developed a minor complication. Physicians typically spend 20 minutes at the bedside and on the patient's hospital floor or unit.

Examples

1. Follow-up consultation of a 65-year-old man, with osteoarthritis who developed abdominal pain upon restarting his NSAIDs following shoulder surgery.

2. AMA/CPT validated example: Follow-up inpatient consultation for a 22-year-old female, established patient, with steroid-dependent systemic lupus erythematosus, arthritis and glomerulonephritis. Patient is reevaluated for loss of consciousness and chest pain.

Follow-up inpatient consultation for an established patient which requires at least two of the following three key components:

1. A detailed interval history
2. A detailed examination
3. Medical decision making of high complexity

Counseling and/or coordination of care with other providers or agencies are provided consistent with the nature of the problem(s) and the patient's and/or the family's needs.

Usually the patient is unstable or has developed a significant complication or a significant new problem. Physicians typically spend 30 minutes at the bedside and on the patient's hospital floor or unit.

Examples

1. Follow-up consultation of a 75-year-old steroid-dependent female with rheumatoid arthritis, who developed new back pain two days following total knee replacement. A complete consultation had been completed one day prior to surgery. Brief examination performed, x-rays, laboratory

and chart also reviewed. Evaluation reveals osteoporosis, compression fractures and osteoarthritis. Patient advised of treatment options and prognosis. Medications instituted accordingly.

2. AMA/CPT validated example: Follow-up inpatient consultation for a 62-year-old female with steroid-dependent asthma, diabetes mellitus, thyrotoxicosis, abdominal pain and possible vasculitis.

Confirmatory Consultations:New or Established Patient

The confirmatory consultation CPT codes 99271-99275 have exactly the same descriptions for history, examination and decision making as the initial inpatient consultation codes (99251-99255), except that they do not include time as a contributing factor. Confirmatory consultation codes can also be used for hospital care (99271-99275).

Emergency Department Services:New or Established Patient

Any physician who provides services to patients registered in the emergency department can use emergency department services codes. Most rheumatologists will not find it necessary to use these codes very often. Their use would be mandated by only three circumstances: (1) the rheumatologist's patient presents in the emergency department; (2) the rheumatologist is called by another physician for a consultation with a new patient; or (3) the rheumatologist is mandated by his hospital to serve as an emergency department physician in order to fulfill a medical staff obligation (this latter obligation would be highly unusual in most areas of the country). If the rheumatologist is called in for a consultation and does not render the emergency treatment, then the outpatient consultation codes (CPT 99241-99245) should be used.

Listed below are the five levels of services that are recognized for both the new or established patient in the emergency department. Examples for each level of service are provided.

Emergency department visit for the evaluation and management of a patient, which requires the following three key components:

1. A problem focused history
2. A problem focused examination
3. Straightforward medical decision making

Counseling and/or coordination of care with other providers or agencies are provided consistent with the nature of the problem(s) and the patient's and/or family's needs.

Usually the presenting problem(s) are self limited or minor.

Example

1. A follow-up visit for a patient receiving daily injections through a heplock. The heplock is functioning well and there is no local infection.

Emergency department visit for the evaluation and management of a patient which requires the following three key components:

1. An expanded problem focused history
2. An expanded problem focused examination
3. Medical decision making of low complexity

Counseling and/or coordination of care with other providers or agencies are provided consistent with the nature of the problem(s) and the patient's and/or family's needs.

Usually, the presenting problem(s) are of low to moderate severity.

Example

1. A patient with known pseudogout calls in after hours and the rheumatologist decides to evaluate the patient's need for joint aspiration. There is no need for any specific treatment when the rheumatologist sees the patient.

Emergency department visit for the evaluation and management of a patient, which requires the following three key components:

1. An expanded problem focused history
2. An expanded problem focused examination
3. Medical decision making of moderate complexity

Counseling and/or coordination of care with other providers or agencies are provided consistent with the nature of the problem(s) and the patient's and/or family's needs. Usually, the presenting problem(s) are of moderate severity.

Example

1. A patient with known pseudogout calls in after hours and the rheumatologist decides to evaluate the patient's need for joint aspiration. The rheumatologist feels that the joint should be aspirated to rule out infection. The joint is aspirated. Phase-contract microscopy reveals positively birefringent crystals and a gram-stain is negative for organisms.

An emergency department visit performed by the same physician on the day of a minor starred (*) procedure such as arthrocentesis may be reported separately if the patient's condition required a significant, separately identifiable E/M service above and beyond the usual preoperative and postoperative care associated with the procedure. This event may be reported by adding the modifier "-25" to the appropriate emergency department visit code (or indicated by 09925), in addition to coding for the procedure. Note: HCFA does not *recognize starred procedures. The procedures eligible for a "-25" modifier are those with zero or 10 post-operative days.*

Emergency department visit for the evaluation and management of a patient, which requires the following three key components:

1. A detailed history
2. A detailed examination
3. Medical decision making of moderate complexity

Counseling and/or coordination of care with other providers or agencies are provided consistent with the nature of the problem(s) and the patient's and/or family's needs.

Usually, the presenting problem(s) are of high severity and require urgent evaluation by the physician but do not pose an immediate significant threat to life or physiologic function.

Example

1. A patient on penicillamine for progressive systemic sclerosis, but without grievous bowel involvement, is seen for diarrhea and mild cramps. She has just returned from a business trip to Mexico and is afebrile. Her abdomen is soft and without organomegaly, her stool is negative for occult blood, and routine blood and urine are negative. She is sent home and will call in the morning unless symptoms worsen.

Emergency department visit for the evaluation and management of a patient, which requires the following three key components within the constraints imposed by the urgency of the patient's clinical condition and mental status:

1. A comprehensive history

2. A comprehensive examination
3. Medical decision making of high complexity

Counseling and/or coordination of care with other providers or agencies are provided consistent with the nature of the problem(s) and the patient's and/or family's needs.

Usually, the presenting problem(s) are of high severity and pose an immediate significant threat to the life or physiologic function.

Example

1. A 47-year-old patient discharged from the hospital five days earlier, on cytoxan 100 mg. per day and prednisone 30 mg. per day, is seen in the emergency department because of abdominal pain and diarrhea. The patient went to a family picnic yesterday and ate chicken which was "slightly undercooked." No one else in the family is ill; the patient is afebrile, bowel sounds are hyperactive and there is slight generalized abdominal tenderness. The white count is 14,000 with a left shift, urine shows 2+ protein, 5-10 W13Cs/HPF, and 50-100 RBCs/HPF (this is similar to the urine at time of discharge). Stool is hemoccult negative, a smear does not show WBCs. Creatinine is 2.1 (it was 2.3 on discharge) and a KUB is negative. The patient's abdominal pain disappears while he is in the hospital. He is sent home on Imodium to be seen in the office the next day.

Critical Care Services

As defined by the AMA CPT manual, critical care includes the care of critically ill or unstable, critically injured, patients who require the constant attention of the physician. (Note: Medicare's definition is critically ill *and* unstable.) The critical care unit is an area where the time required to provide the services is an important determinant of which code to use. CPT code 99291 is used to report the first hour of critical care on a given day. It should be used only once per day even if the time spent by the physician is not continuous on that day. Critical care of less than 30 minutes should be reported with the appropriate E/M service code. CPT code 99292 is used to report each additional 30 minutes beyond the first hour. There are no subsequent follow-up critical care codes. Services for a patient who is not critically ill but happens to be in a critical care unit are reported using subsequent hospital care codes (99231-99233) or hospital consultation codes (99251-99263). For further guidelines, please refer to the AMA CPT manual.

INTRODUCTION TO HEALTH SYSTEMS RESEARCH

THE DEVELOPMENT OF HEALTH SYSTEMS RESEARCH

Why Did HSR Develop?

By adopting of the philosophy and strategies for Health For All, politicians and health staff at all levels are committed to ensuring that *all* people will attain a level of health that enables them to participate actively in the social and economic life of the community in which they live.

Although research has made major contributions to health by providing knowledge of the causes of diseases and by developing the technology to cure and prevent disease and promote health, Health For All is far from being achieved.

Why is there still so much disease that could have been prevented or cured? Because health services by themselves cannot control all of the factors that influence health. Poverty and political systems which either widen or narrow the gap between rich and poor and which promote or neglect the education of girls, for example, influence the health of people. Drought and wars may bring malnutrition and disease with which the health services can hardly cope. While communicable diseases such as smallpox and, to some extent, leprosy may be gradually conquered due to improved environmental conditions and extra effort on the part of the health services, new diseases such as HIV/AIDS may appear which upset the whole health care system and society at large.

This complex of environmental factors – geographical, socio-economic, cultural, political, demographic, epidemiological – not only influences the health of people, it also affects the health services. Countries suffering from poor economics, wars and drought usually have poorly functioning health services as well.

Still, even within less favourable environments, some services function better than others. A very important factor is the quality of information on which policy makers base their decisions. Very often this information is vague or missing. Then decisions on interventions can be completely off track, which means that money is wasted. Basic questions which health policy makers need answered include, for example:

— What are the *health needs* of (different groups of) people, not only according to health professionals but also according to the people themselves? Can shared priorities be agreed upon?

— To what extent do the present *health interventions* cover these priority needs? Are the interventions acceptable to the people in terms of culture and cost, especially to the poor? Are they provided as cost-effectively as possible?

— Given the *resources* we have, could we cover more needs, or more people, in a more cost-effective way? Is it possible to introduce or expand cost-sharing through insurance, to reduce the risk of unexpected high costs, in particular for the economically vulnerable? Could co-operation with the private/ NGO sector be improved? Could donor agencies help solve well-defined bottlenecks in the system?

— Is it possible to better *control the environmental factors* which influence health and health care? Can other sectors help (education, agriculture, public works/roads, etc.)?

These questions cannot be answered without collecting more information through research. That is why, since the end of the 1970's, Health Systems Research (HSR) has been developed.

WHAT IS HEALTH SYSTEMS RESEARCH?

What is Research?

Research is the systematic collection, analysis and interpretation of data to answer a certain question or solve a problem.

Characteristics of research:

— It demands a clear statement of the problem.

— It requires clear objectives and a plan (it is not aimlessly looking for something in the hopes that you will come across a solution).

— It builds on existing data, using both positive and negative findings.

— New data should be *systematically* collected and analysed to answer the original research objectives.

Health research serves two major purposes:

First, basic research is necessary to generate new knowledge and technologies to deal with major unresolved health problems. Second, applied research is necessary to identify priority problems and to design and evaluate policies and programmes that will deliver the greatest health benefits, making optimal use of available resources.

During the past two (or even three) decades there has been a rapid evolution of concepts and research approaches to support managerial aspects of health development. Many of these have been described by specific terms such as operations/operational research, health services research, health management research, applied research and decision-linked research. Each of these has made crucial contributions to the development of HSR (WHO 1990). Health Systems Research is ultimately concerned with improving the health of people and communities, by enhancing the efficiency and effectiveness of the health system as an integral part of the overall process of socio-economic development, with full involvement of all partners.

What is Meant by a Health System?

There are different interpretations of what a health system is. Some give a narrow definition and only consider the different levels of the public health care services as a health system.

The inclusion of the district council, district development committee and village development committee indicates, however, that some 25 years after Alma Ata* it has been widely recognised that local administration and other sectors than the health sector alone carry responsibility for the health of the people in a village, district or region.

Many HSR researchers have a wider perception of health systems. They also include the *private sector*. The private sector has many possible components:

— Non-governmental organization (NGO) care, provided by churches, Red Cross, local NGOs, etc.

— Medical practice by private doctors, nurses, or by quacks who provide injections and drugs without medical training.
— The pharmaceutical sector (licensed pharmacies or unlicensed sellers).
— The large 'non-biomedical' professionalised healing systems (Ayurvedic, Chinese, Unani, homeopathic, chiropractic, etc.)
— Traditional (or folk) medicine, with traditional birth attendants, herbalists and diviners, who may either identify natural or supernatural causes of disease (witchcraft, angry ancestors) and treat patients accordingly.

The Primary Health Care (PHC) approach has broadened the horizon of medical care providers considerably. PHC put individuals and communities in the centre of attention. Individuals providing *self-care* (what mothers and other relatives do to keep children and themselves healthy) and *traditional / folk healers* were accepted as important potential allies of health staff. So were personnel from *other sectors,* which could support health, for example, through the construction of roads, the improvement of education, water, sanitation, and through income generation.

This figure would take different shapes in different societies, but everywhere individuals form part of a *network of family and community members* who are concerned about their health. This network prescribes or advises how to prevent illness and what to do in case of ill health. In many societies, mothers and grand mothers are key figures in early childcare. They determine nutritional and hygiene practices, alert children to dangers, provide care in case of disease, and teach children the basics of self-care.

At the other end of the spectrum, a public authority is responsible for the well being of all people inhabiting its territory. Nowadays governments of states organise public health care and, to some extent, regulate private health care initiatives. Through other social services (e.g., education, social welfare), through laws and taxes and police and army, governments are supposed to assure their citizens the resources to survive and live in peace. Since time immemorial this has been the duty of rulers, although each society has developed its own ways of ensuring 'health for all'.

When in the 1980s many countries were struck by chronic economic crises, the World Bank advocated structural adjustment programmes to reorganise the economies, which relied on market mechanisms rather than on state control with subsidies and protection. The health and educational sectors were inevitably affected and went through a series of reforms that hit the consumer hard. The World Health Organization recognised the need for health reforms, but under the condition that these would leave the goal of HEALTH FOR ALL in tact. It therefore focussed attention on fairness of the system, which should also be affordable to the poor, and at the same time stressed that the system should be responsive to the need of patients for human, respectful treatment.

Functions the Health System Performs: Objectives of the System

Health is expressed as life expectancy by the WHO, taking into account the time lived with a disability of any kind (also due to chronic disease and old age). In the highly industrialised countries of Western Europe, for example, the average life expectancy of men is 74 years, of which 6.5 years are with disability; for women it is 80.8 and 7 years, respectively. In Africa in areas most struck by AIDS, men live now on average only 45.6 years, of which 7.6 years are with disability; for women the respective means are 48 and 8 years. *Responsiveness* to patients' human needs would mean respecting the patient's dignity and autonomy and reducing the fear and shame that sickness brings with it. *Fairness* ideally means financial protection for everyone by payment according to financial capacity. This can best be assured by pre-payment through an insurance system, with fees according to capacity. The insurance revenues are then pooled and costs of care paid from the pool, so that in fact the rich help to cover the treatment of the poor. Unfortunately, such a system is hard to organise in the least developed countries where rural areas harbour mainly poor, but WHO counts on international solidarity and donor agencies for contributions.

The health system comprises both public and private health services but, for the time being, no agricultural, educational or other sectors, however relevant. The first urgency is the *performance* of the health system, which should be as good as possible, given the available means. To reach that aim, WHO set some criteria. Ministries of Health should weigh the public health importance of proposed health actions, set priorities, and thoroughly investigate the cost-effectiveness of different possible interventions to select the highest value for the money. In terms of *resources,* they should strive for a balance between investments, the use made of these investments and their maintenance. For example, if staff members are highly trained but their knowledge is under-utilised, or if buildings, equipment and means of transport cannot be maintained, these investments are highly wasteful. Likewise the services don't function well if there is no money left for consumables such as essential medicines. The patients then have to buy medicines on the private market, out of their pockets and at unnecessary high costs, which the poor cannot afford. Good *oversight* is required to achieve an optimal balance among the different expenses, and it is one of the aims of HSR to provide the policy makers with the relevant data.

Good oversight and 'stewartship' is also required to develop a fair *financing system*. The Ministry of Health is usually the appropriate institution to collect money from taxes and donor agencies to finance the health care system. In the 1980's it became clear that even PHC services could never function adequately with the required coverage (health for ALL) without a contribution from the clients. User fees were introduced in countries that hitherto had provided care free of cost, but this appeared to hit the poor out of proportion despite exemption rules. Hence WHO proposes a more structural solution by introducing prepayment through insurance and pooling of resources, which is beneficial for the poor.

Although the MOH, in many developing countries, is still the principal provider of health care, if it is to achieve the most cost-effective care, it has to consider the use of the private sector and contract services out in cases where this would be cheaper. Consequently, the MOH has to set standards of care and control for deviation in the private sector as well as the public. To have oversight and control is one of the major present day challenges for Ministries of Health.

Specific Questions for Specific Levels of Service

HSR is not only of use to policy makers; at each level managers may have questions that require further research.

Health policy makers may, for example, want to know:

— What are the prospects for voluntary community-based insurance? What would acceptabl contributions for different income groups? Should the pooling of resources take place on a community or national basis?

— How can user-fees be used as an instrument to direct demands for care to the appropriate level?

Managers at district/provincial level may raise questions such as:

— Why is neonatal mortality in certain districts much higher than in other districts?

Hospital directors may ask:

— Why do we have such a high rate of complications during child birth? Are the first-line services available and adequate? Are our own services adequate? Are mothers coming late for delivery and, if so, why?

Managers at village level (village health committees) may want to know:

— How can we assist women with little or no education so that they can effectively recognise the symptoms of pneumonia and go in time to the health centre with their children?

— How much community labour will be required to manage the new water system?

The major objective of HSR is to provide health managers at all levels, as well as community members, with the relevant information they need to make decisions on health-related problems they are facing.

We must be aware that problems at one level of the health system are usually connected with problems or deficiencies at other levels. HSR should address problems from the differingperspectives of all those who are, directly or indirectly, involved. Otherwise we run the risk of coming up with results which only partly explain the problem and which are therefore insufficient to solve it.

PARTICIPANTS IN HSR

It is evident that many issues in health are interrelated and interact with issues in other sectors, such as production, education, the condition of wells or roads, and broader environmental factors. Research in health systems must recognise this. The research skills that are required may need to come from a variety of disciplines, e.g., public health/ medicine, health economics, behavioural and social sciences, and agriculture. Therefore HSR is multi-disciplinary in nature.

Even simple research that is conducted at the operational level may require research skills from different disciplines to provide sufficient and relevant information to support decision-making. Therefore, training in HSR includes relevant aspects from various research disciplines.

Researchers who work in HSR will have to work in a trans-disciplinary way, which means working together as a team throughout all phases of the research. In the process, they need to acquire a basic understanding of the concepts and approaches as well as the potential and limitations of research techniques used in sister disciplines.

HSR, however, is not the concern of scientists alone.

Who should be Involved in HSR?

The participatory nature of health systems research is one of its major characteristics. To ensure that the research is relevant and appropriate, everyone directly concerned with a particular health or health care problem should be involved in the research project(s) focused on it. This may include policymakers, managers from the health and other public services involved, health care providers and the community itself. Their involvement is critical if the research activities are to make a difference:

— If decision-makers are only involved after completion of the study, the report may just be shelved.

— If staff of health and other public services are only involved in data collection and not in the development of the proposal or in data analysis, they may not be motivated to collect accurate data or carry out the recommendations.

— If the community is only requested to respond to a questionnaire, the recommendations from the study may not be acceptable.

— If professional researchers are not involved in the implementation of recommendations, they may have little concern for the feasibility of the recommendations.

The roles that various types of participants will play in the research project will depend on the level and complexity of the particular study as well as its area of focus. Some projects are very complex and may need expertise from several levels, sectors and disciplines. Others may focus on simpler problems and require a more modest set-up. Health personnel may even play a major role in simple studies focusing on practical problems in their own working situations, although their projects may require assistance from researchers with skills in relevant disciplines.

Note: Because of the participatory nature of HSR, in the modules that follow we will use the term RESEARCHER to mean anyone actively involved in planning and conducting the research.

GUIDELINES FOR HSR

Bearing in mind that HSR is undertaken primarily to provide information to support decision-making that can improve the functioning of the health system, we summarise by suggesting some essential guidelines for success:

1. HSR should focus on priority problems in health care.
2. It should be action-oriented, i.e., aimed at developing solutions.
3. An integrated multi-disciplinary approach is required, i.e., research approaches from many disciplines are needed since health is affected by the broader context of socio-economic development.
4. The research should be participatory in nature, involving all parties concerned (from policymakers to community members) in all stages of the project.
5. Studies should be scheduled in such a way that results will be available when needed for key decisions; research must be timely. Otherwise, it loses its purpose.
6. Emphasis should be placed on comparatively simple, short-term research designs that are likely to yield practical results relatively quickly. Simple but effective research designs are difficult to develop but much more likely to yield useful results when needed.
7. The principle of cost-effectiveness is important in the selection of research projects. Program management and operational research should focus, to a large extent, on low-cost studies that can be undertaken by management and service personnel in the course of daily activities. (There is a need for

larger studies as well, however, which may require outside funding and full-time research staff.)

8. Results should be presented in formats most useful for administrators, decision-makers and the community. Each report should include:

   - A clear presentation of results with a summary of the major findings adapted to the interests of the party being targeted by the research.
   - Honest discussion of practical or methodological problems that could have affected the findings.
   - Alternative courses of action that could follow from the results and the advantages and drawbacks of each, formulated with inputs from all parties concerned.

9. Evaluation of the research undertaken should concentrate on its ability to influence policy, improve services and ultimately lead to better health, rather than on the number of papers published.

Thus, an HSR project should not stop at finding answers to the questions posed, but include an assessment of what decisions and activities have evolved from the study.

Bibliography

Bailey R, Weingarten S, Lewis M, Mohsenifar Z. Impact of clinical pathways and practice guidelines on the management of acute exacerbations of bronchial asthma. *Chest* 1998; 113(1):28-33.

Bates DW, Cullen DJ, Laird N, Petersen LA, Small SD, Servi D, et al. Incidence of adverse drug events and potential adverse drug events. Implications for prevention. ADE Prevention Study Group. *JAMA* 1995; 274:29-34.

Bates DW, Spell N, Cullen DJ, Burdick E, Laird N, Petersen LA, et al. The costs of adverse drug events in hospitalized patients. Adverse Drug Events Prevention Study Group. *JAMA* 1997; 277:307-311.

Bowman L, Carlstedt BC, Black CD. Incidence of adverse drug reactions in adult medical inpatients. *Can J Hosp Pharm* 1994; 47:209-216.

Bradshaw BG, Liu SS, Thirlby RC. Standardized perioperative care protocols and reduced length of stay after colon surgery. *J Am Coll Surg* 1998; 186:501-6.

Carter BL, Helling DK. Ambulatory care pharmacy services: the incomplete agenda. *Ann Pharmacother* 1992; 26:701-708.

Choong PF, Langford AK, Dowsey MM, Santamaria NM. Clinical pathway for fractured neck of femur: a prospective, controlled study *Med J Aust* 2000; 172(9):423-6.

Classen DC, Pestotnik SL, Evans RS, Burke JP. Computerized surveillance of adverse drug events in hospital patients. *JAMA* 1991; 266:2847-2851.

Classen DC, Pestotnik SL, Evans RS, Lloyd JF, Burke JP. Adverse drug events in hospitalized patients. Excess length of stay, extra costs, and attributable mortality. *JAMA* 1997; 277:301-306.

Cullen DJ, Bates DW, Small SD, Cooper JB, Nemeskal AR, Leape LL. The incident reporting system does not detect adverse drug events: a problem for quality improvement. *Jt Comm J Qual Improv* 1995; 21:541-548.

Dardik A, Williams GM, Minken SL, Perler BA. Impact of a critical pathway on the results of carotid endarterectomy in a tertiary care university hospital: effect of methods on outcome. *J Vasc Surg* 1997; 26:186-92.

Department of Health and Human Services. Health care financing administration. Fed Regist. 1997; 62.

Dowsey MM, Kilgour ML, Santamaria NM, Choong PF. Clinical pathways in hip and knee arthroplasty: a prospective randomised controlled study. *Med J Aust* 1999; 170(2):59-62.

Dyer CC, Oles KS, Davis SW. The role of the pharmacist in a geriatric nursing home: a literature review. *Drug Intell Clin Pharm* 1984; 18:428-433.

Evans RS, Pestotnik SL, Classen DC, Horn SD, Bass SB, Burke JP. Preventing adverse drug events in hospitalized patients. *Ann Pharmacother* 1994; 28:523-527.

Firilas AM, Higginbotham PH, Johnson DD, Jackson RJ, Wagner CW, Smith SD. A new economic benchmark for surgical treatment of appendicitis. *Am Surg* 1999; 65:769-73.

Folli HL, Poole RL, Benitz WE, Russo JC. Medication error prevention by clinical pharmacists in two children's hospitals. *Pediatrics* 1987; 79:718-722.

Gandhi TK, Burstin HR, Cook EF, Puopolo AL, Haas JS, Brennan TA, et al. Drug complications in outpatients. *J Gen Intern Med* 2000; 15:149-154.

Hanna E, Schultz S, Doctor D, Vural E, Stern S, Suen J. Development and implementation of a clinical pathway for patients undergoing total laryngectomy: impact on cost and quality of care. *Arch Otolaryngol Head Neck Surg* 1999; 125:1247-51.

Hatfield MN, J. The case for critical path. *Cost Engineering* 1998; 40:17-18.

Hatoum HT, Catizone C, Hutchinson RA, Purohit A. An eleven-year review of the pharmacy literature: documentation of the value and acceptance of clinical pharmacy *Drug Intell Clin Pharm* 1986; 20:33-48.

Holmboe ES, Meehan TP, Radford MJ, Wang Y, Marciniak TA, Krumholz HM. Use of critical pathways to improve the care of patients with acute myocardial infarction. *Am J Med* 1999; 107:324-31.

Jenkins MH, Bond CA. The impact of clinical pharmacists on psychiatric patients. *Pharmacotherapy* 1996; 16:708-714.

Jha AK, Kuperman GJ, Teich JM, Leape L, Shea B, Rittenberg E, et al. Identifying adverse drug events: development of a computer-based monitor and comparison with chart review and stimulated voluntary report. *J Am Med Inform Assoc* 1998; 5:305-314.

Johnson JA, Bootman JL. Drug-related morbidity and mortality. A cost-of-illness model. *Arch Intern Med* 1995; 155:1949-1956.

Johnson KB, Blaisdell CJ, Walker A, Eggleston P. Effectiveness of a clinical pathway for inpatient asthma management. *Pediatrics* 2000; 106(5):1006-12.

Kallo G. The reliability of critical path method (CPM) techniques in the analysis and evaluation of delay claims. *Cost Engineering* 1996; 38:35-37.

Kellaway GS, McCrae E. Intensive monitoring for adverse drug effects in patients discharged from acute medical wards. *N Z Med J* 1973; 78:525-528.

Lesar TS, Briceland LL, Delcoure K, Parmalee JC, Masta-Gornic V, Pohl H. Medication prescribing errors in a teaching hospital. *JAMA* 1990; 263:2329-2334.

Mabrey JD, Toohey JS, Armstrong DA, Lavery L, Wammack LA. Clinical pathway management of total knee arthroplasty. *Clin Orthop* 1997; 113:125-33.

Macario A, Horne M, Goodman S, Vitez T, Dexter F, Heinen R, et al. The effect of a perioperative clinical pathway for knee replacement surgery on hospital costs. *Anesth Analg* 1998; 86:978-84.

McDonald CJ. Use of a computer to detect and respond to clinical events: its effect on clinician behavior. *Ann Intern Med* 1976; 84:162-167.

Noedel NR, Osterloh JF, Brannan JA, Haselhorst MM, Ramage LJ, Lambrechts D. Critical pathways as an effective tool to reduce cardiac transplantation hospitalisation and charges. *J Transpl Coord* 1996; 6:14-9.

Pearson SD, Goulart-Fisher D, Lee TH. Critical pathways as a strategy for improving care: problems and potential. *Ann Intern Med* 1995; 123:941-8.

Phillips KA, Shlipak MG, Coxson P, Goldman L, Heidenreich PA, Weinstein MC, et al. Underuse of beta-blockers following myocardial infarction. *JAMA* 2001; 285:1013.

Rumble SJ, Jernigan MH, Rudisill PT. Determining the effectiveness of critical pathways for coronary artery bypass graft patients: retrospective comparison of readmission rates. *J Nurs Care Qual* 1996; 11(2):34-40.

Tett SE, Higgins GM, Armour CL. Impact of pharmacist interventions on medication management by the elderly: a review of the literature. *Ann Pharmacother* 1993; 27:80-86.

Warner BW, Kulick RM, Stoops MM, Mehta S, Stephan M, Kotagal UR. An evidenced-based clinical pathway for acute appendicitis decreases hospital duration and cost. *J Pediatr Surg* 1998; 33(9):1371-5.

Willett MS, Bertch KE, Rich DS, Ereshefsky L. Prospectus on the economic value of clinical pharmacy services. A position statement of the American College of Clinical Pharmacy. *Pharmacotherapy* 1989; 9:45-56.

Willis B, Kim LT, Anthony T, Bergen PC, Nwariaku F, Turnage RH. A clinical pathway for inguinal hernia repair reduces hospital admissions. *J Surg Res* 2000; 88(1):13-7.

Index